D0234825

The Practice of Quality

Donald and Sally Irvine

with a Foreword by
Julia Neuberger

RADCLIFFE MEDICAL PRESS
OXFORD AND NEW YORK

© 1996 Donald Irvine and Sally Irvine

Radcliffe Medical Press Ltd
18 Marcham Road, Abingdon, Oxon OX14 1AA, UK

Radcliffe Medical Press, Inc.
141 Fifth Avenue, New York, NY 10010, USA

All rights reserved. No part of this publication may be reproduced, stored in
a retrieval system, or transmitted, in any form or by any means, electronic,
mechanical, photocopying, recording or otherwise without the prior permission
of the copyright owner.

British Library Cataloguing in Publication Data

A catalogue record for this book is available from the British Library.

ISBN 1 85775 073 X

Library of Congress Cataloging-in-Publication Data is available.

Typeset by Advance Typesetting Ltd, Oxfordshire
Printed and bound in Great Britain by Redwood Books, Trowbridge, Wiltshire

About the authors

Donald Irvine

Donald Irvine was a principal in general practice in Ashington, Northumberland, for thirty-five years. He was a partner at Lintonville Medical Group, a modern teaching and fundholding general practice where many of the ideas described in this book have been tried and tested.

He was also until recently Regional Adviser in general practice at the University of Newcastle upon Tyne. He is a former Secretary and Chairman of Council of the Royal College of General Practitioners and a long-standing member of the General Medical Council. He has written and spoken widely at home and abroad on education and quality in general practice, and has been able to draw on a wealth of experience in developing his ideas and taking these forward.

In 1995 Donald Irvine was the first general practitioner to be elected President of the General Medical Council.

Sally Irvine

Sally Irvine has a background both in management and general practice. After a career in education management and corporate planning with the Greater London Council, she became General Administrator of the Royal College of General Practitioners. Apart from her extensive responsibilities as head of the College's permanent staff, she developed the College's very successful Management Programme, running courses on management appreciation, personnel and appraisal, quality assurance and developmental planning, and providing advice to practices on management development.

She now chairs the Newcastle City Health NHS Trust, which delivers community, mental health and rehabilitative care in the north east of England. She continues with her consultancy and developmental work for individual practices as well as providing seminars and courses for wider groups. Sally has written extensively on organizational and developmental issues in general practice.

In 1994 she was made an Honorary Fellow of the RCGP, and became a Fellow of the Association of Managers in Practice (of which she was President from 1989–93) in 1995.

To Bill Styles,
friend and colleague

Contents

Foreword

In the current ever-changing health care system, maintaining quality in all aspects of health care is of paramount importance. Never has so much been expected of those working in this field and the challenge to general practitioners and the teams of professionals that work with them has never been greater. It is vital that we all understand this task and recognize the educational and developmental requirements it puts upon us all – clinicians, managers and patients alike.

The Practice of Quality is a major contribution to meeting this challenge. It emphasizes putting quality into general practice and into health care as a whole. Each chapter covers a different aspect; such as leadership, working as a team, clinical guidelines, measuring outcomes, and gives helpful, practical advice on tackling the issues and implementing them more effectively.

Areas of particular concern to me are those of accountability, and of growing patient power – consumerism – in health care. This book is aimed both at the practitioner and the lay person – the patient – who wants to get involved in creating better practice, in itself an open approach to patient power. The authors suggest that the forces of consumerism in health care are a good thing, and that patients may decide 'to shop around for health care in future, to go directly to a specialist or try more than one general practitioner rather than use existing pathways …'. This is radical stuff, but it is an excellent example of how they have been prepared to look at all possible eventualities as health care changes over the next decade. The authors point out how health care workers can improve practice, and enjoy their working lives more fully in this rapidly changing environment.

Donald and Sally Irvine have produced a fine work and *The Practice of Quality* must be adopted as a manual by doctors and managers in general practice. I am sure it will become a basic textbook on quality in primary care, and the visionary thoughts of its authors will be shared with its readers. We need to change the way we think about health care, lay or professional; drawing into the discussion those who use the service, those who provide it, and those who purchase it on the public's behalf. In discussing how we can do better in the new scheme of things there is no better place to start than this book.

Julia Neuberger
Chair Camden and Islington Community Health Services NHS Trust.
Member of the GMC, the Medical Research Council, and a vice-president of
the Patient's Association

January 1996

Acknowledgements

The ideas set out in this book are the result of many years' experience in and around general practice for both of us. Our first thanks must go to the many practices that have formed the bedrock of that experience, both in a consultancy capacity and as professional colleagues.

The book is also the result of many long discussions with many distinguished colleagues and friends, both medical and non-medical. We are grateful to them all for their patience and the insights they have given us.

We are particularly grateful to Hilary Haman, Michael McKendrick, Peter Mitford and Michael Pringle for reading the final text and giving us such helpful and constructive comments.

We are very indebted to the six colleagues who contributed the case studies that form Chapter 15. Their willingness to share their experience and reflections is much appreciated, and our thanks too go to their partners and practice teams for agreeing to reveal themselves in this way.

Finally, as usual, none of this would be possible without the unstinting help and support of Angela McGlaughlin at the Postgraduate Institute for Medicine at the University of Newcastle upon Tyne and Anne Whensley, Sally's personal assistant.

Introduction

In the UK general practice is often equated with primary health care because almost every person in the country is registered with a general practitioner. The general practitioner is the person to whom people usually turn first when they are unwell. Today general practice is steadily evolving as a system of primary health care based on the primary health care team. It is extending its traditional role in providing continuing personal care for the individual patient, and adding to this the new capacity to know about and improve the health status of the group of people who make up the registered list. This inclusive concept of general practice, embracing personal and population medicine, has the potential to become the central pillar of primary health care, which itself is now being seen as the foundation of the National Health Service (NHS). Our book is about this kind of general practice.

QUALITY – THE KEY TO SUCCESS

The book reflects our conviction that the key to success for all practices lies in the promotion of a culture that involves quality in all its dimensions. We believe that good quality care results when practice teams are confident, knowledgeable and skilled, are able to work together effectively, can see where they want to go and can ensure that they achieve their objectives. Our conviction stems from our first-hand knowledge and experience of general practice gained from practising it, observing it, teaching it and advising on it. Our background may help to explain why the emphasis is heavily on the people who make up the practice team.

The book is divided into five parts, each dealing with an important element in the achievement of such a way forward. The first part (Chapters 1 and 2) is about why a practice needs to be aware of the context in which it functions, especially of the factors at work in the wider world and the NHS which are bringing about change. It is essential for a modern, quality-minded practice to be aware of such factors, and of their possible impact on general practice. Awareness means that a practice is less likely to be taken by surprise, and is more likely to be able to anticipate the implications of change. From awareness comes a sense of direction – a fundamental element of leadership and therefore of quality practice.

The second part (Chapters 3–5) looks at the concept of quality, what it is and how it can be measured and assessed in general practice. It is an introduction to the theoretical foundation that is the starting point for understanding how the various practical ways and means of assuring and improving quality fit together.

In the third part (Chapters 6–13) the key components of management in practice are discussed: an understanding of how power is distributed, the role of leadership and teamwork, how to plan ahead and how to make sure that a practice has the people with the right knowledge and skills. The underlying theme is the need to manage people effectively, be they partners, professional colleagues or other members of the team. Effective management is the key to the successful implementation of good-quality care.

Practitioners and their practices are becoming more explicitly accountable for their competence and performance. The fourth part (Chapters 14 and 15) looks at the system of professional self-regulation within which they work, and how this is evolving through certification and accreditation to assure patients that they are in safe hands.

Finally we will present our concluding thoughts. But we will keep these to the end!

OUR READERS

The book has been written for the growing number of practice teams that would like to take their practices forward with quality very much in mind. It should be of particular interest to the growing number of general practitioners, nurses and practice managers who are assuming special responsibility for policy development, quality assurance and quality improvement within their own practices. Although lightly referenced for easy reading, further references are given for those who wish to explore the subject in more depth. Anonymized examples, based on our experiences, are used freely since front-line practitioners seem to find these useful to relate to and compare with their own experience. The major case studies in Chapter 15 have been written by the practice members themselves.

The book will also be of interest to health service managers, particularly those in the new health authorities who are commissioning, developing and managing primary care, and to executive and non-executive directors of health authorities and trusts who are interested in learning more about primary health care and its future. Furthermore, patients and other users will find it helpful as they explore the various means by which they can contribute in a structured and systematic way to quality in general practice.

In the general practice of tomorrow quality will be everybody's business.

Quality Practice – Being Aware of the Context

1

General practice in a changing world

God and the doctor we alike adore,
But only when in danger, not before,
The danger o'er, both are alike requited,
God is forgotten, and the doctor slighted

John Owen (1560?–1622)

A PRIMARY CARE-LED NHS?

Primary health care, and general practice, are in a period of unprecedented change. The Alma Ata declaration, published by the World Health Organization, described primary health care as 'the first level of contact between people and the national health system', and as the entitlement of all citizens.[1] Lee[2] sees primary health care as a set of activities, a process, a level of care and as a strategy for organizing the health care system as a whole. Starfield[3] describes it as: 'first contact, continuous, comprehensive and co-ordinated care provided to populations undifferentiated by gender, disease or organ system'.

In the NHS it consists mainly of general practice, the community nursing services including the community psychiatric services, the professions allied to medicine, dental and optical services and many others. Until now it has been separate and distinct from the secondary care provided by specialists in hospitals.

Despite the often stated importance of primary health care, the emphasis and the investment in the first 50 years of the NHS has nevertheless been on hospitals and hospital care. Primary care has been seen – and has often seen itself – as the poor relation, the rather messy and unsexy part of the service through which patients pass on their way to hospital or to which they return after specialist treatment. The term 'gatekeeper', or even 'gateopener', has had pejorative overtones.

Now this is no longer the case. The ageing population, increasing prevalence of chronic degenerative disease, advances in the science and technology of medicine and spiralling costs of health care together emphasize the value of keeping patients as far as possible in their home environment – and out of expensive hospital beds. It is factors such as these that are driving the search for better ways of organizing and coordinating primary and secondary care. As a result, government and the NHS[4-6] have started the so-called *strategic shift* from secondary to primary care, towards a primary care-led service.

One thing is already clear. The extent to which primary health care services are able to establish themselves as the reliable foundation of the future NHS will depend substantially on four things:

1 providing a range of high-quality personal health services in the community which people need and want, provided that resources are available
2 evolving professional attitudes, skills and ways of working that result in effective and efficient care for patients which people value
3 achieving improvements in the health status of the practice population
4 giving value for money.

Primary health services that satisfy these criteria, and demonstrate that they achieve them, are most likely to survive in an increasingly competitive world. Effective quality assurance and quality improvement are essential for ensuring success.[7,8]

General practice: the basis of primary care

General practice is now seen by policy-makers as the logical basis for primary health care. Recently, the Department of Health[9] summarized the reasons why this should be so (Box 1.1).

Box 1.1   WHY GENERAL PRACTICE SHOULD BE THE CORE
OF PRIMARY CARE[9]

- the registered list of patients generally covers 99% of the population
- general practice is understood and accepted by the public
- teamwork is strengthened
- the coordination of care is made smoother
- the sharing of records is made easier
- communication is improved, and
- the health care professionals involved can help to build up accurate pictures of local needs

---

THE CHANGING WORLD

The acceptance of this core role by general practice makes it vital that individual practices regularly take time to appraise the significance for them of the factors for change in medicine and the wider world. This kind of reconnaissance provides the basis for planning ahead. In the remainder of the chapter, and in the next, we have done our own crystal ball gazing, our own scanning the horizon. We hope this will give readers a feel for what this involves when they come to make their own predictions and perform their own analysis.

A brief note of caution. Change usually has its downside as well as its benefits. And an opportunity for one practice may be seen as a threat by another. This is why it is so important that each practice carries out this kind of exercise for itself; moreover, the exercise should be repeated regularly, because facts, and the perceptions of their importance, change. Opinion and forecasts like ours can only ever be an aid. The factors driving change in general practice are shown in Box 1.2.

Box 1.2   FACTORS DRIVING CHANGE IN GENERAL
PRACTICE

- demographic change
- changing patterns of disease
- advances in medical science/technology
- the microchip revolution
- social change
- costs of health care
- more accountability

Demographic change

The most striking demographic change in the UK will be the shift in the balance of the population towards a higher proportion of elderly people as death rates fall and more of us live longer. There are now over 4000 centenarians in Britain compared with 300 some 40 years ago. In 1991, 807 000 people were aged over 85; by 2015 there will be 1.5 million. However, 8% of those aged 65–75 are disabled, rising to 40% for the over-85 age group.[10] Increase in age brings with it a greater likelihood of dependency and disability due to illnesses such as arthritis, stroke, dementia and chronic circulatory and respiratory disease. The significance of this change in population balance lies in the momentum it will generate for more care in the community. For every general practice the ageing population will therefore be a major factor in planning and implementing practice services.

Changing patterns of disease

In the UK chronic degenerative diseases have replaced communicable diseases as major causes of death. However, viral, bacterial and parasitic mutations are continuous and can occur extremely quickly. They can effectively defeat existing medical technology, as meningitis outbreaks and AIDS have shown.

The causes of death are changing. For example, between 1951 and 1991, while deaths from communicable diseases reduced dramatically, the proportion of deaths attributable to accidents and violence rose substantially. The proportion of total deaths from cancers (particularly for women) and circulatory diseases also rose sharply.[11]

As practices become more used to assessing the health status and health needs of their registered populations, so they will become more accustomed to measuring mortality and morbidity within their own micropopulations. The aggregate of these will describe the important characteristics and trends in the health of local communities. Such practice-derived data will therefore become the basic building blocks in determining local health policies and priorities in the early part of the coming decade.

Advances in medical science/technology

Scientific and technological advances and innovation in medicine proceeds at a breathtaking pace. Doctors who began practising, say, 40 years ago could not have envisaged, for example, the striking dimensions of the coming revolution in transplant surgery, the virtual elimination of killing and disabling infections such as measles and poliomyelitis and the nature of the advances in the medical and surgical treatment which have changed – and continue to change – the focus of care between general practice and hospital.

- Forty years ago most births took place at home. Domiciliary obstetrics were therefore a core function of general practice. Today most births are in hospital, and intranatal care in general practice has almost disappeared.
- Forty years ago morbidity from duodenal ulcer was high, with frequent emergency admissions for intensive medical treatment and, invariably, surgery. Today open-access gastroscopy and contrast media radiology, and the effectiveness of drug treatment, have made the management of duodenal ulcer dyspepsia a general practice function.
- Until recently, angina was diagnosed and managed largely in general practice unless it became severely uncontrolled. Today more frequent hospital referral is required because current technology enables precise assessment of the pathology, and angioplasty and coronary artery bypass surgery in appropriate cases improve the quality of life.

- Forty years ago patients with diabetes mellitus were looked after by general practitioners and specialists working almost independently of each other. Now they are managed on a 'shared care' basis. They attend their practice for routine supervision, much of it by the practice nurse. Specialists confine themselves to well-defined circumstances when the patient's condition requires their additional expertise. This is a pattern of care for many of the major chronic illnesses.

Looking ahead all the evidence points towards even more technical development in medicine.

- With the growth of minimally invasive therapy and day-case surgery, it is likely that within ten years fewer than one-third of patients undergoing surgery will have to stay in hospital overnight.
- The revolution in molecular biology, exemplified by the Human Genome Project, will have profound effects on our ability to predict, prevent and perhaps in time treat genetically influenced disease.[12]
- There is the prospect of a new generation of designer drugs targeted at, for instance, some of the cancers and dementia.
- There is likely to be even more extensive use of organ transplants and the introduction of artificial organs and tissues and refined prostheses engineered to give patients substantial control.[11]

General practice is always likely to remain a low-technology user in medicine compared with the subspecialties, which tend to require ever more sophisticated equipment. However, even so-called low technology can be quite sophisticated, as the following examples show.

- The use of multifunctional desk-top laboratory analysers is now being evaluated in general practice.
- General practitioners have immediate access to packaged very high technology (in the form of drugs) that extends their ability to treat and manage serious illness.
- The general practitioner's emergency bag will include a defibrillator as standard equipment.
- There will be open access to more hospital-based diagnostic technology, such as exercise tolerance testing, endoscopy examinations and more advanced radiology.

The microchip revolution

Medicine and health care are information-based and information-driven disciplines. Huge databases are already being assembled, linked and accessed internationally, and yet made user-friendly for individual health professionals through radio and satellite communications.

This information technology revolution, which has hardly touched the NHS yet, will almost inevitably bring about dramatic change across all health services. Some examples certain to affect general practice include:

- hand-held computers, which will become as indispensable as stethoscopes for tomorrow's general practitioners and community nurses
- more effective data handling and transmission among practices, between practices and hospitals and between practices and patients in their homes. This will be achieved through facsimile transmission and direct computer links, such as the information superhighway
- practice appointments systems that will be computerized, so freeing up receptionists to give personal help to patients
- access in the consulting room to local, national and international clinical databases through the Internet
- the science of informatics, significantly extending the clinical role of general practitioners by giving them immediate access in the consulting room to unsolicited computer prompts and information they consciously seek.[13] Purves[14] describes ways in which doctor-requested information may be used for:

  1 differential diagnostic support
  2 clinical epidemiology
  3 browsing information when defining a clinical problem
  4 accessing computerized guidelines
  5 intelligent presentation of information to the patient

- videophone links between doctor and patients at home, making videophone follow-up and 'advice' consultations popular, resulting in fewer patients needing to attend surgery for these purposes
- telediagnosis and video-conferencing between general practitioners and specialists, altering current patterns of referral, with less travelling to specialists by patients. By the year 2000, remote consultations will be commonplace in the image-based specialties such as dermatology and radiology.[15] For example, remote links have already been established between practices on the Isle of Skye and hospital dermatologists in Inverness, with a reduction in outpatient attendances of 75%
- electronic records, encoded on a smart card, which will give patients physical charge of their case notes in an easily transportable form.

These illustrations give a flavour of the huge impact that information technology is likely to have on the work of general practice. It will take the concept of 'one-stop' medicine a stage further. Box 1.3 summarizes the areas where the information technology revolution will have an impact on health services including general practice.

Box 1.3   AREAS AFFECTED BY THE MICROCHIP REVOLUTION

- the medical consultation
- the ways in which patients use health services
- the nature and location of buildings required for health care
- the distribution and organization of work among health professionals
- the way in which their knowledge and skills are deployed to optimum advantage
- better information to patients

Social change

Social factors influence health and play an important part in determining the demand for health care (Box 1.4).

Box 1.4   SIGNIFICANT FACTORS AFFECTING DEMAND FOR HEALTH CARE[16]

Some key social trends
- ageing population
- reduction in community spirit
- more crime and violence
- more fragmented families
- smaller households
- rising levels of education
- rising expectations
- changing social attitudes to health

Some key economic trends
- increasing national wealth
- less heavy industry
- more women at work
- more part-time employees
- more people switching careers
- higher unemployment
- wider income disparities
- public spending capped

There are three areas in particular where social change is having an impact on health and health care.

Health and illness

Patterns of health and illness are influenced by social circumstances, environment and lifestyle. There is a relationship, for example, between the economic status of patients, the quality of their housing and their health.

Equally, environmental influences (such as air pollution) and lifestyle habits (such as smoking, drug abuse) also directly affect survival rates and quality of life.

Consumerism

The health reforms of the early 1990s sought to make the NHS more responsive to patients. In doing so they reflected the growing power of consumerism in the UK and in the western world. The Patient's Charter is one manifestation.

The NHS, like the other social services established after World War II as part of the welfare state, has had a strong provider bias. Consumerism, albeit multifaceted, is forcing a reorientation of the NHS, including general practice, so that it becomes centred on the patient, rather than on the provider. Practices are being asked to ensure that the surgery is welcoming and friendly, with facilities for children, nursing mothers and the disabled. Individual patients are seeking more information about their condition, sight of their records and to be told about the effectiveness of the measures taken to diagnose and treat their complaints. Patients and health authorities expect practices to survey opinion among the registered population to find out whether people are generally satisfied with their care, and where improvements can be made.

This trend is likely to continue as the users of health care become better informed and use the new-found powers which information technology gives them.

- Patients may decide, whatever doctors and the NHS say, that they prefer to shop around for health care in future, to go directly to a specialist or try more than one general practitioner rather than use existing pathways, so circumventing the referral system, particularly if they have smart cards.
- Even if the referral system is retained, patients may well want more say about which doctors they should go to, or which hospitals they should attend, on the basis of published league tables of performance to which they have ready and independent access.

Health professionals

Nor are health professionals themselves immune from social change. For example, as a new balance between male and female doctors is established in medicine, part-time working and job sharing are increasing, as in other areas of employment. Furthermore, doctors are mirroring society in being less inclined to work unsocial hours. There is pressure to create more space within the working week for family and other non-medical activities. These changes all have implications for the size and deployment of workforce and the organization of work in general practice.

Costs of health care

It is self-evident and widely acknowledged that the capacity of medicine to provide now outstrips society's ability to pay for all that is possible. Within the next decade the debate about the ethics and mechanics of rationing health care will become more focused and more urgent, and will involve general practice as much as any other part of the NHS.

Fundholding and commissioning are already bringing home the costs of care and forcing doctors and nurses to try and think more clearly than ever before about the relationship between cost and quality, how it is to be managed and what their roles should be.

More accountability

The twin motors of consumerism and cost containment are resulting in growing pressure on health professionals to become more accountable for their work. There are three inter-related dimensions. Patients seek more direct accountability within the doctor–patient relationship as the balance of power shifts towards patients, as said earlier. Second, there is growing pressure for more accountability to peers, informally through clinical audit (Chapter 4) or more formally through the licensing and certificating bodies of the health professions (Chapters 14 and 15). Third, there is pressure for more account-ability from management, an unsurprising development in a health service that is coming to be based on the principles of 'managed care' (Chapter 6).

CONCLUSION

As this chapter shows, general practice is having to adapt to the huge forces for change. Against this background, and more by chance than by design, general practice based on the registered population is in a position to provide the ideal base for the sort of health care that is emerging. In adapting and changing, a different kind of practice will develop, as we explore in the next chapter.

REFERENCES

1   World Health Organization (1978) *Alma Ata 1977. Primary Health Care.* Geneva: WHO UNICEF.

2   Lee P R (1994) Primary care tomorrow: models of excellence. *Lancet;* **344**: 1484–6.

3   Starfield B (1984) Primary care tomorrow: is primary care essential? *Lancet*; **344**: 1129–33.

4   Secretaries of State for Health, Social Services, Wales, Northern Ireland and Scotland (1987) *Promoting Better Health: the Government's Programme for Improving Primary Health Care* (Cmn 249). London: HMSO.

5   Secretaries of State for Health, Social Services, Wales, Northern Ireland and Scotland (1989) *Working for Patients* (Cmn 555). London: HMSO.

6   NHS Executive (1994) *An Accountability Framework for GP Fundholding: Towards a Primary Care Led NHS.* London: NHSE.

7   Clinical Outcomes Group (1994) *Clinical Audit in Primary Health Care.* London: NHS Executive.

8   Royal College of General Practitioners (1994) *Quality in Practice.* Policy Statement No. 2. London: RCGP.

9   NHS Executive (1993) *Nursing in Primary Healthcare: New World, New Opportunities.* London: NHSE.

10 Oram J, Millard P H (1995) How to care for an ageing population. Letter to *The Times*, February 24.

11 Appleby C, Ham C (1995) *The Future of Health and Health Care Services: a Report for Healthcare 2000.* Birmingham: Health Services Management Centre, University of Birmingham.

12 Watson J D (1990) The human genome project: past, present and future. *Science*; **248**: 44–9.

13 Coiera E (1995) Medical informatics. *British Medical Journal*; **310**: 1381–6.

14 Purves I N (1995) Computerised guidelines in primary health care: reflections and implications. In *Health Telematics for Clinical Guidelines and Protocols* (eds Gordon C, Christensen J P) Technology and Informatics 16. Amsterdam: IOS Press.

15 Wright R, Loughrey C (1995) Teleradiology. *British Medical Journal*; **310**: 1392–3.

16 National Association of Health Authorities and Trusts (1994) *Closer to Home: Healthcare in the 21st Century.* Research Paper No. 13. London: NAHAT.

2

A different kind of practice

To achieve the true aim and end of general practice – its mission to preserve a humane medicine for persons – many of its current restrictions, uniformities, boundaries and monopolies must also come to an end

Marinker (1994)[1]

GENERAL PRACTICE TODAY

All practices today provide primary and continuing care. In addition, all practices can influence the nature and range of secondary care through their engagement with health authorities in the commissioning of care. Fund-holding practices are able to purchase some secondary care, hold their own drug budgets and contract directly with community trusts for district nurses, health visitors and other community-based services.

General practice has a huge workforce. There are about 35 000 general practitioners in the UK working in some 10 000 practices based mainly on small partnerships. They are supported by some 50 000 receptionists, secretaries and practice managers, and they work with the whole-time equivalent of around 50 000 nurses, including district nurses, health visitors, practice nurses and community psychiatric nurses.[2]

Changes in general practice over the last 20 years

General practice has been the subject of an accelerating evolutionary change, especially in the past ten years. The main movements are shown in Box 2.1.

The move from reactive to planned care began with preventive services, but now has extended to the management of chronic care in many practices and all care in some. Individualism among general practitioners is deeply rooted in the culture and is the source of much strength as well as something of an Achilles heel. The strength of this individualism helps to explain

---

Box 2.1   MOVEMENTS IN GENERAL PRACTICE

Traditional practice		**Modern practice**
Reactive care	⟶	Planned care
Individualism	⟶	Teamworking
Provider focus	⟶	Patient focus
Personal responsibility	⟶	Collective responsibility
Implicit (variable) standards	⟶	Explicit standards
Single model	⟶	Flexible provision

why the team approach to collective responsibility in partnerships and in the wider practice is only just getting under way. The extent to which this change is made successfully will, more than any other factor, determine how well general practices can adapt to life in the modern world. Movement towards explicit standards and flexibility in the provision of practice-based services are recent phenomena, and are responses to the changes described in Chapter 1.

There seem to be four general conclusions from these movements:

1 the move from traditional to modern practice implies major changes in attitude and ways of working for health professionals
2 new skills are needed to negotiate change successfully
3 there remains considerable variation since some practices have changed completely, some are still wholly traditional and most are probably somewhere between
4 the rate of change from traditional to modern practice appears to have accelerated as a result of the 'new contract' and fundholding.

A consensus is now emerging about what the features of general practice should be[3-5] and therefore what patients can expect today (Box 2.2).

Box 2.2   ESSENTIAL FEATURES OF GENERAL PRACTICE TODAY

Patients are entitled to expect:

* safe, effective personal care
* easy access to services
* choice of health professionals
* continuity of care
* good coordination with other services
* care at home when needed

These features embody much of the traditional general practice that patients like and which will be so appropriate as the basis for primary health care in future. General practice has to be local and evenly distributed within the populations served, so ensuring the continuation of easy access to care that patients consistently say is of great importance to them. Home care remains an important feature for those who are temporarily or permanently housebound because of illness; people like and expect it. However, the content of services is already beginning to expand and diversify as the boundary between what is done in hospital and what is done in the community becomes more fluid and blurred. More flexible arrangements for providing continuity of care, especially in relation to out-of-hours care, are now under consideration.

The persisting problem of wide variations

Variations in the structure of health services and in the patterns of care provided by health professionals are a feature of health services here and abroad. This is particularly true of general practice, where very wide variation in clinical practice has been and is still a significant problem. The nub, it would seem, is the lack of any clear and generally agreed definition of the range and level of clinical responsibilities that general practitioners should undertake. This historically very open-ended approach to the job has resulted, at one extreme, in care of a very sophisticated kind and at the other in a level of care that is little more than basic triage, with only the very simplest problems being dealt with in the practice setting.

Variations may be seen in all major clinical activities. Prescribing, the use of hospital radiology and laboratory services, referral to specialists, record keeping and doctor-initiated return consultations are among the commonest and most significant areas. The causes are multifactorial, but the common thread linking all seems to lie in the behaviour of individual clinicians, in particular how and why they come to their decisions about diagnosis and patient management.

Much of the drive towards greater accountability in general practice, especially the exercise of greater clinical accountability through measures such as clinical audit, is directed to reducing the size of this variation. In particular, there are both professional and management initiatives that aim to reduce and ideally eliminate those variations that are the result of poor practice, hence the growing interest in quality assurance and quality improvement.

It is very important to distinguish between variation that is not only legitimate but indeed to be welcomed, because it meets patient preferences and because there are legitimate clinical options, and that end of the spectrum of clinical practice where patients are put at risk without justification. In seeking to focus on this latter aspect of variation, the concepts of clinical effectiveness, clinical appropriateness and evidence-based practice should be helpful.

CHANGES IN PRACTICE

We turn now to consider the main areas where we think the changes described in Chapter 1 will have their greatest impact. These are summarized in Box 2.3.

Box 2.3   PROBABLE IMPACT OF CHANGE FACTORS IN GENERAL PRACTICE

- expansion in range and content of services for individual patients
- development of the population-based dimension of practice
- focus on patient-centred care
- drive for improved health outcomes
- development of evidence-based practice
- more effective teambuilding
- changes in the organization of work
- diversity of contracting arrangements
- blurring of boundary between primary and secondary care
- teaching and research

Three general points need to be made at the outset. First, it is becoming clear that change in health care is becoming the norm rather than the exception. Later in the book (Chapter 9) we consider how practices can try to avoid being taken by surprise by change.

Second, there is evidently going to be much more flexibility in the way primary care is provided and organized in future. There will be much greater emphasis on diversity to try and reflect local needs and preferences and encourage experiment and innovation.

Third, clinicians will be under increasing pressure from patients, peers and managers to demonstrate that they are maintaining their clinical skills at an optimum level, and expanding these where there may be advantage to patients.

Personal care: the range and content

Tomorrow's patients are more likely than ever to choose their practice based on what it can offer them and their families. The more that can be provided locally the better, provided that the quality is right.

The range of services is steadily expanding, especially since fundholding opened up new opportunities. Thus, for example, some practices now offer dietetic advice, counselling, chiropody, physiotherapy, complementary therapies and similar supporting services. Specialist consultations may be provided by visiting consultants. A few practices have beds attached. The expansion in the range of services has tended to be contract driven. Thus, for example, changes in the payment structure for immunization, cervical cytology and other preventive procedures led to more of these being under-taken. And the recent development of minor surgery in general practice was contract led.

Changes in the depth of care provided within general practice are also accelerating. The concept of the general practitioner with extended clinical skills – the doctor with a special clinical interest – is likely to become widely established as higher training is introduced. Some of the early higher training proposals include a clinical component, such as ophthalmology, dermatology and ear, nose and throat (ENT). In tomorrow's practice genetic counselling and greater medical support for patients with significant psychiatric illness are coming onto the agenda. We have already mentioned in Chapter 1 how the forthcoming use of computer-assisted diagnosis should enable general practitioners to go further in unravelling patient problems themselves and in consultation with partners with a special interest.

In expanding the range and depth of services, it will be important for general practices to be able to resist having 'dumped' on them tasks for which they are unprepared and for which they thus have neither the time, skills nor other resources necessary to do well. The practice of tomorrow will find it vital to have the kind of management arrangements that enable it to retain control and so ensure that desired new services are actually feasible. Quality assurance will be essential if extended clinical services are to reflect the standards of care which the public will expect, and if practices are to protect themselves against pressures for expansion in situations where quantity could become the enemy of quality.

The population dimension

The system of patient registration, unique to the NHS, has always held the potential of combining services for individual patients with the practice of population medicine. However, for many years that potential lay largely unrealized, partly because of the relatively low priority given to preventative medicine, but mainly because of the lack of means for abstracting and aggregating data simply and cheaply from the clinical record.

Today the public health dimension is assuming much greater importance. Hart[6] foreshadowed this development in the late 1980s. His ideas were given greater prominence in the new general practice contract, which offered in-centives for preventive and health education interventions. Looking forward, it is now recognized that the registered list provides the basis for profiling the health status of a practice population, and for assessing patients' health needs and expectations.

The addition of a public health function to general practice has been greeted with some misgivings, which have been most cogently explained by Pratt.[7] There are general practitioners who feel that the new emphasis on trying to improve the health care of a defined population is severely eroding individual patient care, not least because some procedures required under the new contract have been of questionable clinical value. Fundholding practices are also experiencing the tension between individual and population medicine, as they try to reconcile the needs of individual patients with the allocation of finite resources at the practice level.

In reality, personal care and population care in general practice are not alternatives, nor are they mutually exclusive. On the contrary, both are desirable and important functions that can aid and facilitate the other. Any conflict between them should be eased as practice management and practice computing become more sophisticated. Thus, morbidity recording, data abstraction and analysis and the assessment of health needs and expectations on an on-going basis should become more straightforward, integrated into a practice's management arrangements and therefore more economical in terms of the time and effort that clinicians have to spend on it.

Focus on patient-centred care

Earlier we mentioned consumerism as a powerful force for change. Dennis[8] published a study outlining new approaches to consumer feedback in general practice. She foreshadowed the role of patients in developing practice guidelines and standards. She recommended that patients should be asked by survey, clinical audit and other means to say how their practice works for them, in terms of access, in the way that they are handled when they seek help and about the results of the care they receive. The involvement of patients in standard setting and performance monitoring in a systematic way within each practice is coming.[9,10]

The key question now is how to make consumer involvement work successfully. There are reports of practices commissioning surveys of patient expectation and satisfaction based on representative samples of the registered list. The patient participation group is another approach. Yet other practices are appointing one or two patients as the equivalent of non-executive directors to their partnership or practice management boards. All practices are now being encouraged to establish their own internal complaints procedures. And, outside the practice, consumer feedback through community health councils and other local groups is being actively sought both by the new health authorities and by practices themselves.

It is equally clear that, in the renegotiation of the boundary between health professionals and the people for whom they provide care, the health professionals will rightly expect patients as consumers to use a practice's services responsibly. They will expect them to assume greater responsibility for those aspects of their health over which they have direct control, such as smoking, drinking, exercise and other lifestyle habits that influence health.[11]

Drive for improved health outcomes

The last decade has seen a major movement in health care throughout the western world, directed to developing measures of the *outcome* of care, that is the effects of care on patients. We explain this further in Chapter 3.

The problem in general practice is that good measures of outcome are difficult to devise. Many presenting symptoms never crystallize into recognizable clinical entities. Chronic conditions, by definition, run their course over long periods of time, making it difficult to attribute change in a patient's condition to single health care interventions when many other potentially significant variables are present at the same time. And viral illnesses, which are so common in general practice, are self-limiting, and so it is not worth spending time and money trying to measure outcome in such cases.

Nevertheless, the outcomes movement is gathering pace in primary care, and forward-looking practices will want to know what measures are in use now, what will be coming on-stream shortly and how these might best be used in the practice setting. For example, mortality is still a valuable indicator of outcome when assessing the effectiveness of care in patients with meningococcal meningitis. Similarly, functional measures such as school attendance have a clear role in assessing outcome in conditions such as asthma in children.

Development of evidence-based medicine

The search for care that confers the best possible benefit at the lowest possible cost has led to growing interest in the concept of *evidence-based* practice, expressed practically in clinical guidelines (Chapter 5) and as a means of improving clinical problem solving.[12] Evidence-based practice is about using tests and treatments which research has shown should confer benefit, that is lead to an improvement in the patient's condition. The principle of justification in clinical decision making, whereby doctors must be prepared to explain the rationale of their clinical decisions, is as old as medicine itself and is built into the profession's ethic. The new developments in evidence-based practice may extend the principle a step further as they try to bring some degree of formality to the process.[13] The movement has been given focus in this country by the establishment of the Centre for Evidence-Based Medicine at Oxford.

It has to be acknowledged that many clinical actions are of dubious value if one looks for definitive scientific proof that they lead to a beneficial improvement (improved outcome). Thus, evidence-based practice is also about discontinuing investigations and therapies that have no proven value, that is are not clinically effective.

As evidence-based practice gathers momentum, it is important for clinicians and managers to keep in mind the self-evident fact that there are important aspects of care that have obvious value but which cannot be measured formally, and so might be held to be scientifically inappropriate. The amount of time spent listening to patients' complaints and offering explanation and support is an obvious example. On such important but subjective aspects of care, clinicians should be fully prepared to use their clinical judgement.

However, the evidence-based approach to clinical care should lead to more decisions which are clinically effective. Clinical effectiveness describes interventions that improve outcome. And, arguably, clinical effectiveness will be linked in future with the idea of cost-effective care by introducing an economic dimension, as Donabedian[14] argued long before the idea became fashionable. So here, in the substance of the outcome movement, clinical effectiveness, clinical appropriateness and evidence-based medicine, we begin to see a cluster of new elements to clinical practice that general practitioners now need to master.

The move to teamwork

The combined effect of the multiple factors driving change, especially the need to find the most cost-effective way of doing things, is forcing a re-examination of traditional patterns of working. Moreover, modern health care increasingly implies teamworking, not just between doctors but between doctors and other health professionals. This poses a problem for those health professionals, particularly doctors, whose education and upbringing has focused almost wholly on the integrity of the doctor–patient relationship, with little regard to the effectiveness of working relationships with colleagues.

It is now over ten years since the Royal College of General Practitioners proposed a framework for teamworking in general practice.[15] It reflected back to an even earlier time when district nurses and health visitors were first attached to general practice, and a supporting staff of receptionists, secretaries and others began to assist in the operation of general practice. Yet recent research from Sheffield bears out the widely held view, based on experience and anecdotal evidence, that teamworking in general practice is in fact something of a myth.[16] It is only recently that the medical profession has begun to grasp the importance and significance of teamwork in modern health care and has started to seek ways of making teams work (Chapter 10).[17]

Changes in the organization of work

Closely linked with effective teamworking is the issue of skills mix.[18] A major redistribution of work is now under way across all disciplines in the practice team, with much more emphasis on the nursing input.[19] Since Stillwell's[20] pioneering work on the role of nurse practitioners, more nurse practitioners are being introduced to UK general practice. For example, in a development in the Northern and Yorkshire Region future nurse practitioners are being taught to assess patients with apparently minor illness, referring on to the general practitioner only those who have potentially more serious complaints that need further investigation.[21] And practice nurses and nurse practitioners are already well established in their clinical role in the management of chronic illness.

Similarly, almost the whole of preventative medicine and health education may be carried out more effectively by nurse practitioners than by doctors, not least because of their proven record of complying closely with clinical protocols and guidelines. Were there to be no change in the content of general practice as we know it now, it would thus be quite conceivable to envisage a switch in the balance of labour deployment between nurses and doctors, in favour of nurses. At the same time general practitioners are themselves likely to take on new functions, to become perhaps more like general physicians practising in the community, creating a new balance between generalists and specialists.

Diversity of contracting arrangements

Yet another consequence of the drive for high quality and lower cost is the new interest in the use of differing contracting arrangements. A recent survey has shown that, for example, a substantial minority of younger doctors would prefer salaried employment to working as an independent contractor.[22] Greater flexibility in contracting arrangements is likely to reflect more closely the particular needs of local communities and their providers.

Possible future configurations of contracting within general practice are shown in Box 2.4.

Traditional contract

It is virtually certain that, for the foreseeable future, many general practitioners will want to continue to be employed on the present nationally negotiated contractual arrangement whereby there is a personal agreement between doctor and health authority. This may be particularly appropriate and relevant for single-handed practices and for smaller practices in which

---

Box 2.4 POSSIBLE FUTURE CONTRACTING
CONFIGURATIONS

- current contract with individual doctor
- free-standing group – contract with practice
  - without fund
  - with fund for practice-based services only
  - with fund for practice-based services plus selected secondary care
  - total fundholding
- wider provider – NHS trust or new health authority provides the service

---

the arrangement does not interfere unduly, because of size, with collaborative working arrangements within a practice. Locally negotiated contracts may develop within a national framework.

Practice contracts

Today's fundholding practices are the prototype of tomorrow's free-standing group practices in which any practice, regardless of size, could contract with a health authority to provide a specified range and quality of service for a defined population, at an agreed cost. The role of the fundholding practice, or whatever its successor is called, as a provider would become pre-eminent, with additional elements added to the budget for hospital care where desired. Fundholding practices would become, in effect, small NHS trusts operating their own 'mini health service'. The current centrally negotiated contract could become one of a series of contracts, which, together, could provide the practice with an income weighted to reflect the health needs of its population, from which all staff and services would be paid. The practice could enjoy considerable autonomy as to how it organized patient care and would be judged by its results. It might or might not choose to purchase secondary care.

The NHS Executive[23] now recognizes three types of fundholding:

1 community fundholding, for practices of a small size, limited to the practice's own services and some community services
2 standard fundholding, which in addition to practice services includes some surgery and outpatient care, and specialized nursing
3 total purchasing for practices that are a locality purchaser of all hospital and community health service care for their patients.

The wider provider

The third major variant is the so-called *wider provider*, whereby a trust or health authority becomes the employer of doctors and nurses and begins to function as a provider in its own right. Several experiments have already begun. For instance, the health authority in Liverpool is directly employing some general practitioners in the inner-city area to ease the problems of quality in practice there. Newcastle City Health, a large mixed trust, has recently taken on a local general practice at the doctors' request; the practitioners have salaried contracts on the basic consultant scale.

It can only be a matter of time before more hospital trusts decide to offer primary health care either by establishing links with neighbouring practices or by employing doctors and nurses directly or by a combination of these arrangements. Similarly, ambulance and paramedic trusts may collaborate with general practitioners and/or community trusts in the organization and delivery of out-of-hours care.

Blurring of the boundary between primary and secondary care

Mention has already been made of the inherently fluid nature of the boundary between secondary and primary care. However, the involvement of general practice in the purchasing of care is having a profound effect.

All practices are now in a position through either the direct purchasing or the indirect commissioning of care to influence the shape and quality of secondary care. This purchasing/commissioning function would appear to be opening up a new dialogue between primary and secondary care, and in the immediate future this is likely to involve more contact between clinicians in these two sectors.

Five prominent consequences are likely to flow from these activities. These are listed in Box 2.5.

Box 2.5   CONSEQUENCES OF GENERAL PRACTICE
                   COMMISSIONING OF CARE

- access for patients to secondary care is likely to be improved in terms, for instance, of reduced waiting times
- better criteria, expressed in the form of clinical guidelines and protocols, are likely to provide a more rational basis for referral between primary and secondary care, and back again
- there is likely to be better use of resources, with less duplication of effort, particularly in outpatients
- practices are likely to become the monitors and external assessors of the quality of secondary care for patients
- through purchasing and commissioning, practices may have a new role as advocates for resources on their patient's behalf

---

Teaching

About one in ten practices today has a teaching function, notably with vocational registrars. However, the use of general practice as a basic source of clinical experience for all the disciplines that make up the primary health care team is now beginning to be seen as a further consequence of the shift from primary to secondary care. An example of how the range of teaching services could be extended is shown in Box 2.6.

Box 2.6   THE MULTIDISCIPLINARY TEACHING PRACTICE

- basic medical education for medical students
- general clinical training (pre-registration year)
- vocational training for general practice
- experience in general practice for future specialists
- continuing medical education for general practitioners

   Medical

- basic training for nurses
- special training for health visitors, community nurses, practice nurses
- community psychiatric nurses and nurse practitioners
- continuing education for all nurses in the community

   Nursing

- training and continuing education of practice managers
- training and further education of receptionists and other practice support staff

   Administrative and secretarial

There are quality implications for this development. Since general practices acquired teaching responsibilities 20 years ago, teaching practices have been subject to external professional controls exercised through the selection and reselection of arrangements that still operate today. This framework is generally acknowledged to have been more successful than any other in helping to bring about desired change and innovation, and is likely therefore to form the basis for the wider management of the multidisciplinary teaching practice of tomorrow.

THE CORE FUNCTIONS OF GENERAL PRACTICE

We have spent some time exploring the probable impact of the change factors in the NHS on general practice. Against the background of these changes and their consequences, the core functions of future general practice are set out in Box 2.7.[24]

Box 2.7   THE CORE FUNCTIONS OF FUTURE PRACTICE

- to provide care of good quality to individual patients
- to improve the health of the practice population
- to secure secondary care of good quality for individual patients, when required
- to promote learning, teaching and research

THE PRIME IMPORTANCE OF QUALITY

Each of these functions brings us hard up against the need to ensure quality. A major international trend is the movement towards the adoption, wherever possible, in health care of explicit standards, and to the use of systems of monitoring that enable practitioners and managers to determine whether these are adhered to and therefore achieve the benefits expected. In the UK the science of clinical guidelines construction and use is still in its infancy, and effective performance monitoring is still time-consuming and expensive because of the absence of the appropriate information technology. However, this can be expected to change quite quickly as the revolution in information technology proceeds.

The consequences of this for health professionals will go well beyond standard setting and performance monitoring. Such consequences include the need for a reappraisal of concepts of professional accountability, in particular the boundaries between health professionals, managers and the users of health care to which we have already referred. General practice will be expected to seek high standards of practice and care through a process of incremental continuous improvement, to assure patients that they are receiving good care and to protect patients from poor care.

We consider the principles, approaches and methods of quality assurance both in theory and in practice in the next part.

REFERENCES

1   Marinker M (1994) *The Eighth Bayliss Lecture, 1994: The End of General Practice*. London: Private Patients Plan.

2   Audit Commission (1992) *Homeward Bound: a New Course for Community Health*. London: HMSO.

3   Royal College of General Practitioners (1996) *The Nature of General Medical Practice*. Reports from General Practice 27. London: RCGP.

4   Joint Working Party of Royal College of General Practitioners and Welsh General Medical Services Committee (1994) Patient care and the general practitioner. *British Medical Journal*; **309**: 1144–7.

5   Gray D P (1992) *Planning Primary Care*. Occasional Paper 57. London: RCGP.

6   Hart T (1988) *A New Kind of Doctor*. London: Merlin Press.

7   Pratt J (1995) *Practitioners and Practices: a Conflict of Values?* Oxford: Radcliffe Medical Press.

8   Dennis N (1991) *Ask the Patient: New Approaches to Consumer Feedback in Good Practice*. London: College of Health.

9   Clinical Outcomes Group (1994) *Consumer Involvement Initiatives in Clinical Audit and Outcomes: a Revision of Developments and Issues in the Identification of Good Practice*. London: DoH.

10   National Consumer Council (1992) *Quality Standards in the NHS: the Consumer Focus*. London: NCC.

11   Dunstan G R (1994) *Ideology, Ethics and Practice*. Second John Hunt Memorial Lecture. London: RCGP.

12   Rosenberg W, Donald A (1995) Evidence-based medicine: an approach to clinical problem-solving. *British Medical Journal*; **310**: 1122–6.

13   Evidence-Based Medicine Working Group (1992) Evidence-based medicine: a new approach to teaching the practice of medicine. *Journal of the American Medical Association*; **268**: 2420–5.

14   Donabedian A (1966) Evaluating the quality of medical care. *Milbank Memorial Fund Quarterly*; **44**: 166–203.

15   Royal College of General Practitioners (1983) *Promoting Prevention*. Occasional Paper 22. London: RCGP.

16   West M, Poulton B, Hardy G (1995) *New Models of Primary Health Care: the Northern and Yorkshire Region Micro Purchasing Project*. Leeds: NYRHA.

17   Berwick D M, Enthoven A, Bunker J P (1992) Quality management in the NHS – the doctor's role. *British Medical Journal*; **304**: 304–8.

18   Heath I (1994) Skill mix in primary care. *British Medical Journal*; **308**: 993–4.

19   Marsh G N (1995) Establishing a minor illness nurse in a busy general practice. *British Medical Journal*; **310**: 778–80.

20   Stillwell B (1991) Defining a role for nurse practitioners in British general practices. In *Directions in Nursing Research* (eds Wilson-Barnett J, Robinson S). London: Scutari Press.

21   Alberti G (1995) *Nurse Practitioner Project*. Research and Development, Northern and Yorkshire RHA, unpublished.

22   General Medical Services Committee (1992) *Your Choices for the Future: a Survey of GP Opinion*. London: BMA.

23   National Health Service Executive (1994) *Developing NHS Purchasing and GP Fundholding*. EL (94) 79. Leeds: NHSE.

24   Irvine D H (1993) General practice in the 1990s: a personal view on future developments. *British Journal of General Practice*; **43**: 121–5.

Quality and Standards

3

Quality – the theory

Quality is in the eye of the beholder

Quality is an absolute. It is like beauty, justice and truth, a 'Holy Grail' always to be aspired to and never to be achieved. We can all recognize quality, especially where there is a defined, single end product such as an item of clothing or a new car. Quality may also be relatively easily perceived in a service. We may think, for example, that as parents we can distinguish good education from less good education, and we know when the service in a restaurant is excellent, good or awful. Although the quality of a specific service is less tangible than that of a manufactured product, we as consumers usually have little difficulty in making a judgement that we can explain to others.

The quality of health care is a more complicated matter. Modern health care comprises a complex raft of activities and services even within a relatively small organization such as a general practice. And there is no well-defined customer. Is it the patient who is clearly the ultimate beneficiary of care? Or is it the health authority with whom the health professionals are in contract? Is it the tax-payer? Or is the fundholding general practitioner a customer when commissioning specialist services from hospitals on behalf of the practice population?

Ovreteit[1] describes this multifaceted situation as the 'complex customer'. Among these customers there will be different ideas about quality, and within each group individuals will vary. For example, patients are not homogeneous, as Case Study 1 shows.

To complicate matters even further, some activities in health care can delight the patient yet, for example, offend the tax-payer because they may be seen as not essential. Some cosmetic plastic surgery procedures come into this category. Similarly, there are patients who would like to be prescribed an antibiotic for every cold, not a view of quality their doctors would share.

Case Study 1

Dr Jones had been in practice for 25 years, with no record of patient complaints against him. He had a strong following in the rural community where he worked with two much younger partners, Drs Brown and White. He tended to see the more elderly female patients and the adult males. He had a rather brusque manner, which his supporters saw as being 'very straight'. His two young partners were rather appalled by the way he treated patients but, as there were no obvious complaints, they did nothing.

However, the newer younger families in the village were not so thrilled by his approach, and began to express the view that he was rude and uncaring. One day, when Dr White was unexpectedly off sick, Dr Jones came in on his half-day off to do most of her surgery. Several younger women he saw were put off by his manner. When he told one young girl to pull herself together and stop complaining about her dysmennorhoea, the girl's mother decided to report him to the FHSA for rudeness and lack of care. He sought support from several of his devoted patients, who could not understand why the girl's mother was making a fuss.

Little wonder, then, that concepts of quality in health care have been so difficult to pursue. Quality of health care is very clearly multidimensional.

THE COMPONENTS OF QUALITY CARE

Avedis Donabedian, the doyen of quality assessment in health care, used the idea of *goodness* to link three closely inter-related components.[2] First, there is what he called the 'goodness' of technical care. There is, he argued, a value attaching to technical care that is proportionate to its effectiveness, that is to its expected ability to achieve the greatest improvement in health status that science, technology and clinical skill can offer at any moment in time. Technical quality, defined in this way, may thus be equated broadly with the contemporary concept of *clinical effectiveness*.

Second, goodness can be applied to interpersonal relationships. The relationship between the patient and the doctor, nurse or other health professional is the most obvious aspect but, in modern general practice, team relationships are as important. This dimension of quality would thus embrace, for example, the care and sensitivity with which a consultation is managed, the effectiveness of communication between doctor and patient, respect for patients' privacy including the protection of information held about them, and, at a team level, the closeness of working relationships.

Donabedian's third component of quality refers to the goodness of the amenities and the environment of care. Is the surgery reasonably accessible for mothers with children? Is the building warm and the reception welcoming? Are there adequate facilities for disabled patients? Is there an appointments system and does it work as it is supposed to do? The amenities are not critical to clinical effectiveness, but they can help indirectly by putting patients at their ease, and by creating working conditions for staff that are conducive to effective performance.

In the UK Robert Maxwell took Donabedian's ideas an important stage further when he identified six core components of quality.[3] These have stood the test of time and are widely used today within the NHS. Later he attached questions to each component to help define further the meaning of quality.[4] These components and the related questions are reproduced in Box 3.1.

Box 3.1   QUESTIONS THAT HELP TO DEFINE AND EXPAND
THE LABEL 'QUALITY'[4]

Effectiveness   Is the treatment given the best available in a technical sense, according to those best equipped to judge? What is their evidence? What is the overall result of the treatment?

Acceptability   How humanely and considerately is this treatment/service delivered? What does the patient think of it? What would/does an observant third party think of it? ('How would I feel if it were my nearest and dearest?') What is the setting like? Are privacy and confidentiality safeguarded?

Efficiency   Is the output maximized for a given input or (conversely) is the input minimized for a given level of output? How does the unit cost compare with the unit cost elsewhere for the same treatment/service?

Access   Can people get this treatment/service when they need it? Are there any identifiable barriers to service – for example, distance, inability to pay, waiting lists, and waiting times – or straightforward breakdown in supply?

> **Box 3.1:** *continued*
>
> Equity   Is this patient or group of patients being fairly
>   treated relative to others? Are there any identifiable
>   failings in equity – for example, are some people
>   being dealt with less favourably or less appro-
>   priately in their own eyes than others?
>
> Relevance   Is the overall pattern and balance of services the best
>   that could be achieved, taking account of the needs
>   and wants of the population as a whole?

Both Maxwell's and Donabedian's ways of looking at quality may be compared with the components of quality described by a World Health Organization (WHO) Working Group on Quality,[5] which suggest that quality must
reflect at least the following four concerns:

1 performance (technical quality)
2 resource use (economical efficiency)
3 risk management (the identification and avoidance of injury, harm or
   illness associated with the service provided)
4 patient (or client or customer) satisfaction.

Blending the components

There is clearly a substantial measure of consensus in each of these
definitions, and indeed in similar formulations from other writers. And, as we
have already noted, differing views on quality will be provided by patients,
practitioners and purchasers of care. Different groups of individuals within
each of these categories will produce subtle differences in emphasis, blending
the components to describe what they mean by quality. The US Joint
Commission on the Accreditation of Healthcare Organizations[6] concluded
that, in general terms:

- quality for patients means predominantly responsiveness, politeness and
  relief from symptoms or an improvement in function
- quality for practitioners means primarily technical skill, freedom in care
  provision and desired outcome
- quality for the purchasers of care means first and foremost efficiency and
  savings.

Until recently blending the components of quality was seen as relatively
straightforward because, certainly in the NHS, doctors and nurses have
tended to think that their perspective of quality should prevail. Their
perspective is indeed important because it will help to determine the strength
of their commitment, which is critical to effective clinical performance.

However, in recent years, as we have seen in earlier chapters, patients, as organized consumers, have begun to assert their right to have their say not only in determining what the standards of care might be, but also in assessing the results of that care for themselves. It is common experience, for example, that patients are becoming increasingly critical of difficulties they may encounter in getting to see their own general practitioner, or of being kept waiting for their appointment at the surgery, as shown in Case Study 2.

Case Study 2

A practice partnership had just completed a major rebuild of its premises, of which the practice members were justly proud. Just after the opening, a solitary old man was sitting in the new modern waiting area, where he was joined by one of the partners, Dr Skinner.

'Well, Bill, what do you think of it?' Dr Skinner asked.

To her surprise, Bill replied, without batting an eyelid,

'I'll tell you whether it is any better when I see whether you start your surgery on time now!'

The Patient's Charter[7] is a good example of the formal expression of consumer will through parliament. Managers (and government) have also become far more independently assertive on quality matters, seeking by managerial action to establish their own agenda of what constitutes good quality and in particular what gives good value for money. Indeed, in the new NHS health authorities see themselves as acting on behalf of patients, there to find out what patients need, what they want, and what they think of what they already get, as the starting point of the commissioning process.

The debate on quality is continuous at all levels in the health service because of the inherent tensions between the main players, and because of the ever-shifting nature of health care and the social environment within which it is provided. The concepts of quality described above provide us with a starting point. These, however, are of themselves insufficient to furnish a basis for assessing, and thus ensuring and improving, quality.

A FRAMEWORK FOR ASSESSING QUALITY

Donabedian gave us a framework for measuring and assessing quality with his now classic triad of *structure*, *process* and *outcome*.[8] This triad is widely used by clinicians, health service management and patients' organizations in the UK because it provides the most rational basis for the assessment of quality. It is summarized here.

Structure

Donabedian used the word *structure* to describe the physical features of health care. Structural characteristics would thus comprise, for example, the surgery premises, the number of doctors, nurses and other practice personnel, the range and type of equipment, the records and all the many other features which in combination make up the primary health care environment. Donabedian argues that good structure, that is a sufficiency of resources and proper systems design, is probably the most important means of protecting and promoting the quality of care.

The earliest studies of general practice tended to emphasize structure, not least because of its visible relationship with resources. These studies were concerned primarily with the numbers of doctors and nurses, the physical characteristics of practice premises and the presence or absence of items of equipment. Comparisons were made between different kinds of practices, practices in different areas and so on. More structure tended to be equated simplistically with better care. Today structural characteristics are regarded as rather blunt instruments for indicating quality even though they can be measured easily. Structural characteristics may increase or decrease the probability of good clinical performance, but the relationship between structure and a doctor's performance (which is about process) is tenuous. For example, the presence of a cervical speculum (structure) in the treatment room does not guarantee that all doctors will always use it (process). Nevertheless, if there is no speculum, that part of the examination cannot be done.

Nevertheless structure is an important part of the environment of care. Major deficiencies in practice premises, staffing and equipment make the provision of good care more difficult, as the patients and health professionals of many inner city practices know only too well.

Process

Donabedian defined the massive complex of clinical interactions and activities between doctors and their patients, and indeed any other 'doing' activities within a practice, as the *process* of care. Process characteristics therefore reflect, for example, examinations done, prescriptions written, tests carried out, patient advice given and the countless other transactions between health professionals and patients or between health professionals themselves. Information about the nature of process may be obtained either by direct observation, that is by sitting in with another doctor in the consulting room;

watching video consultations; or, most commonly, by a review of data in the patient's records, which may allow a more or less accurate reconstruction of what has gone on in the consulting room, at the patients' bedside or in the surgery reception.

An assessment of the process of care, that is what the doctors and other members of the practice team do, is a primary objective of peer-led audit. A judgement on the quality of a particular part of the process will depend upon what is known about the relationship between the characteristics of that part and the consequences for the health and well-being of individuals and of society. The characteristics of the processes of care and their consequences are therefore, Donabedian argues, determined partly by the state of medical science and technology at any given time and partly by norms that govern the management of the relationship between health professionals and patients.[2] Inevitably, these may change as a result of scientific advance or an alteration in societal values, as illustrated in the examples set out in Box 3.2.

Box 3.2   EXAMPLES OF PROCESSES AFFECTED BY CHANGES IN SCIENCE AND SOCIAL ATTITUDE

- The prescription of a drug (process) which is regarded as good practice in one year may be seen as potentially hazardous in the next because new facts come to light about the drug's side effects. Thalidomide and Opren are well-known examples.
- In Britain in recent years, patients collectively have begun to assert that their doctors are excessively paternalistic in the doctor–patient relationship. Now doctors are reacting by adjusting their attitude and approach (process) as more patients insist on more information about their care, and more say in what will happen to them.

In other words the quality of the process of care is defined primarily as normative behaviour, in which the norms derive from either the science of medicine or the ethics and values of society. And norms reflect quality only in the extent to which they contribute to valued consequences.

Linking process with quality is therefore attractive to health professionals. It simplifies matters for them, not least because process describes what they do. They feel reassured that they are giving good-quality care if they believe that they are doing their best within the 'conventional wisdom' of medicine, that is what is considered at the time to be good practice. This is irrespective of whether such practice can be shown ultimately to result in a definable, beneficial effect on the health status of patients, that is whether it is clinically effective.

Outcome

Donabedian defines *outcome* as the changes in a patient's current and future health status that can be attributed to past health care. Outcomes are therefore the ultimate indicators of health. They are concerned with the effects of care. For example:

- does the patient live or die?
- does the patient get better?
- is the patient left with residual handicap or impairment of physical or mental function?
- are there clinical complications?

Outcome is therefore the final arbiter of quality. There are numerous possible approaches to the definition of outcomes. Donabedian preferred a broad definition of health, so that good outcomes would include improvement in social and psychological functions as well as improvement in the more usual physical and physiological aspects. He also included patient attitudes such as satisfaction, health-related knowledge acquired by the patient and health-related behaviour.

There has been much debate about the relative validity, reliability, feasibility, accessibility and cost of process and outcome measures as expressions of the quality of health care. In reality, process and outcome variables may merge one with another in a linear progression. The term *intermediate outcome* is therefore used to describe measures that may be regarded as either process or outcome, depending upon where they are between the input and output ends of an imaginary continuous line (Figure 3.1).

Structure ⟶ Process ⟶ Intermediate outcome ⟶ Definitive outcome

Figure 3.1   The relationship between structure process and outcome.

The value of intermediate outcomes is that they predict, or are assumed to predict, definitive outcome. And they are invariably easier to measure than definitive outcomes, as illustrated in Case Study 3.

Outcomes of health care can be conceptualized in different ways. One easily remembered classification identifies the five Ds: death, disease, disability, discomfort and dissatisfaction.[9] Examples of some types of outcome measure and their possible applications in general practice are shown in Table 3.1.

Developing valid measures of outcome is one of the major research challenges in general practice today. The field is more circumscribed than one might think because, for instance, there is no point in trying to devise measures for the huge volume of self-limiting infections which present in general practice, nor is it always possible to define quantifiable outcomes for such important attributes in general practice as 'tender loving care'.

Case Study 3

The Moore Practice ordered its activities (*the process of its care*) so as to achieve a 100% immunization rate against whooping cough. The ultimate measure of success (*definitive outcome*) was to be the elimination of the occurrence of new cases of the disease, and the mortality and morbidity associated with it, in the practice population.

Clearly, for the practice measuring the immunization rate revealed part of the process chain. However, the achievement of a defined immunization rate could also be seen as an *intermediate outcome*, and worthwhile on its own, because in this case it would be a good predictor of *definitive outcome*. If the practice managed to immunize most people at risk, then there would be fewer cases of whooping cough in the practice population (*definitive outcome*). Relying on counting cases of whooping cough to measure a definitive outcome would therefore never achieve a realistic result – indeed it could take forever – because the very point of immunization is to eliminate the disease.

Lastly, in recent years in Britain it has become fashionable, both in the medical profession and in health management circles, to promote the view that only outcomes count. This fashionable tendency has to be resisted, for in its way it is as untenable as the proposition that only process or only structure should count. Real improvements flow when there is a judicious balance between these three, with particular emphasis on the relationship between process and outcome.

Aspects of structure, process and outcome which describe good quality are all capable of being defined as measurable entities to which data may be attached. These descriptions become the criteria and standards from which practice policies and clinical guidelines and protocols are constructed.

CRITERIA AND STANDARDS

The items of data which together describe a patient's condition and the care given are often called elements. Their huge number alone requires selectivity if they are to have practical value as the building blocks for quality assessment.[10] A criterion is one of these elements carefully selected to measure and assess a clearly defined aspect of care, such as the recording of the patient's temperature, pulse or blood pressure, and therefore the performance of the doctor providing the care. Criteria should be discrete, clearly definable and

Table 3.1   Examples of some aspects of the outcome of care and possible applications in general practice

Aspect of outcome	Example	Application
Death	Case fatality from meningitis	Review of past management for evidence of delay in diagnosis or inappropriate emergency treatment
Functional capacity	Freedom from acute asthma in childhood; no absence from school	Comparing treatment regimens between partners, and between practices
Cure	Skin cancers	Comparing practitioners for evidence of early diagnosis
Clinical complications	Wound infection rates following minor surgery	Comparing general practices (including nursing care)
Health status	Herd and personal immunity against rubella in females of childbearing age	Comparing immunity status in practice populations
Patient satisfaction	Feeling of satisfaction with the continuing management and care of patients with chronic diseases such as diabetes and hypertension	Postal surveys and interviews to compare practices and practitioners

precisely measurable, reflecting aspects either of structure, process or outcome which are specifically related to quality.[2] Criteria are best developed by professionals relying on expert opinion in their own field and on the scientific literature.[11]

The term standard is used to describe the precise numerical level of a criterion of care. If a criterion of the process of care is, for example, the recording of the measurement of blood pressure, then the statement that 90% of all patients who see a doctor for any reason should have their blood pressure taken within a six-month period would be a standard of the process of care.

We can put criteria and standards together to build up a series of statements describing good clinical practice. These process criteria and standards are called clinical guidelines. They are thus preformed recommendations issued for the purpose of influencing decisions about health interventions.[12]

Each of the criteria which make up a guideline will have been chosen because of its relevance to quality in the particular situation concerned (Case Study 4).

Case Study 4   Elements into guidelines[13]

Two general practitioners and two paediatricians constructed a guideline describing the diagnosis and management of acute abdominal pain in children under 11 years of age. The statement contained 406 criteria identified as indicating good practice. Some of these criteria were regarded as more important than others. Thus, for example, the criterion identifying rebound tenderness in the right iliac fossa carried with it the essential requirement to refer to hospital. However, there were rather more criteria developing the diagnosis and the plan of management, for which a particular course of action was considered to be highly desirable but not essential. These criteria offered the doctor guidance and so introduced a greater degree of flexibility, but there was still the assumption that departures from such criteria would be exceptional. Beyond this, there were many more criteria for which the doctor had a number of legitimate options. Indeed, all remaining criteria that were not mandatory or near mandatory were options.

This distinction between mandatory, almost mandatory and optional criteria and standards follows closely that described by Eddy,[14] who classified criteria according to the weight of scientific evidence linking them to desired clinical outcome.[15] He described 'standards' as appropriate care which should be followed in all circumstances with no flexibility for the clinician; 'guidelines' should be followed in most circumstances but with some flexibility in some circumstances and 'options' are so flexible as to provide virtually no guidance at all. Clinical guidelines, so derived, are becoming one of the most important tools in modern practice. We say more about them, therefore, in Chapter 5.

CONCLUSION

Quality in health care is indeed a complex business. In this chapter we have attempted to display the essence of the principles and concepts involved, but in doing so acknowledge fully that some subtleties and nuances have been lost through oversimplification.

However, readers will be able to use their own imagination, and place their own interpretation upon matters when we move on in the next chapter to the practical realities of implementation.

REFERENCES

1   Ovreteit J (1992) *Health Service Quality.* Oxford: Blackwell.

2   Donabedian A (1980) The definition of quality: a conceptual exploration. In *Explorations in Quality Assessment and Monitoring.* Vol.1: *The Definition of Quality and Approaches to its Assessment.* Ann Arbor: Health Administration Press.

3   Maxwell R J (1984) Quality assessment in health. *British Medical Journal;* **288**: 1470–2.

4   Maxwell R J (1992) Dimensions of quality revisited: from thought to action. *Quality in Health Care;* **1**: 171–7.

5   WHO Working Group (1989) The principles of quality. *Quality Assurance in Health Care;* **1**: 79–95.

6   Joint Commission on the Accreditation of Health Care Organizations (1989) *Quality Assurance in Managed Health Care Organizations.* Chicago: JCAHO.

7   Secretary of State for Health (1991) *The Patient's Charter: Raising the Standard.* London: HMSO.

8   Donabedian A (1966) Evaluating the quality of medical care. *Milbank Memorial Fund Quarterly;* **44**: 166–203.

9   Lohr K N (1988) Outcome measurement: concepts and questions. *Inquiry;* **25**: 37–50.

10 Horder J, Marinker M, Pendleton D *et al.* (1986) Terminology of performance review. In *In Pursuit of Quality* (eds Pendleton D, Schofield T, Marinker M). London: RCGP.

11 American Medical Association Advisory Committee on PSRO (1974) Task force on guidelines of care: PSROs and norms of care. *Journal of the American Medical Association;* **229**: 166–77.

12 Lomas J, Haynes R B (1988) A taxonomy and clinical review of tested strategies for the application of clinical practice recommendations: from 'official' to 'individual' clinical policy. *American Journal of Preventative Medicine;* **4**: 77–94.

13   North of England Study of Standards and Performance in General Practice (1990) *Final Report: Setting Clinical Standards Within Small Groups.* Newcastle upon Tyne: Health Care Research Unit.

14   Eddy D M (1990) Clinical decision making: from theory to practice: practice policies – what are they? *Journal of the American Medical Association;* **263**: 441–3.

15   Irvine D H, Donaldson L (1993) Quality and standards in health care. *Proceedings of the Royal Society of Edinburgh;* **101B**: 1–30.

4

Quality – the practice

*Achieving and maintaining good quality primary health care is
most likely to happen where the practitioners who make up each
practice unit are themselves committed to the philosophy, principles
and methods of quality assurance and quality improvement*

Clinical Outcomes Group (1995)[1]

To have any practical effect, the concepts and theoretical models for describing quality which we discussed in the last chapter have to be translated into instruments and mechanisms which will give patients certain guarantees about quality.

The term *quality assessment* has been defined as 'the comparison of care against predetermined standards'.[2] Quality assurance goes one step further than quality assessment, requiring action to be taken on any deficiencies revealed by such assessment.[3] Moreover, it is a planned activity:

> the formal and systematic exercise of identifying problems in medical care delivery, designing activities to overcome the problems, and following up to ensure that no new problems have been introduced and that corrective actions have been effective.[4]

REGULATION OR IMPROVEMENT?

Today it has become usual to look at quality assurance in two ways, each complementing the other. One is long established. This is *quality by inspection*, and characterizes the regulatory function which requires that bad apples are removed. The certification of professional standards, and (practice) accreditation come into this category, and are discussed fully in Chapter 14. The strength of the regulatory approach is that it provides clear external standards, which may be embodied within a professional, statutory or contractual framework, which if effectively applied will give the public some fundamental guarantees on performance. The weakness is that it can encourage a minimalist approach. Health professionals, being human, will in the main be content to jump through predetermined hoops, and limit themselves to that, without striving to go further.

The concept of continuous quality improvement – and total quality management – has its roots in industry. W Edwards Deming and J M Juran were American citizens invited at the end of World War II to advise the Japanese on statistical process control in engineering.[5] They, and Ishikawa, were the architects of the quality revolution which has given Japanese industry such a commanding lead in the world economy.

Deming, in his now classic monograph,[6] identified '14 points' that he considered crucial to quality improvement. These are set out in Box 4.1, together with our commentary on what each means for practice. The nub of quality improvement, Deming said, is that 'it all has to do with reducing variation'.

Box 4.1   IMPROVING QUALITY: DEMING'S 14 POINTS

Deming	**Our comment**
1 Create constancy of purpose	Commitment Leadership Sense of direction Teamwork
2 Adopt the new philosophy	The attitude of mind that seeks improvement across the entire spectrum of patient care
3 Cease dependence on inspection	Build quality in Get it right first time
4 Cease awarding business on the basis of price alone	Establish longer term relationships between purchasers and providers so that quality and strategic development can happen Applies especially to fundholders
5 Improve continuously and for ever	Does a practice have coherent systems for organizing and delivering care? Attitude of 'could we do better?' Strategy required for sustaining interest and commitment

Box 4.1: *continued*

6	Institute training and re-training on the job	Careful attention to the personal professional development – and hence performance – of all practice staff is a 'must'
7	Adopt and institute leadership	Deming believes that most quality problems are the responsibility of management
		We agree. Doctors, as the 'proprietors' of a practice, have an imperative leadership responsibility in helping to identify and solve problems
8	Drive out fear	Depends on leadership
		In good practice teams people will feel they can speak out when something is wrong, or could be better, without fear of retribution or ridicule
9	Break down barriers between staff	In practices, like the NHS, people tend to work in their own professional boxes. Yet good patient care demands effective collaboration – team again!
10	Eliminate slogans, exhortations and targets from the workforce	Mission statements in the practice business plan extolling 'excellence' and 'quality' in every other sentence are useless without the data, systems and skills that help ordinary people in the practice team to overcome their everyday frustration with notes that get lost, surgeries that do not seem to run on time, etc.

Box 4.1: *continued*

11	Eliminate numerical quotas for workers and numerical goals for managers	Numbers are an essential part of quality assurance, especially clinical audit. It is how they are used that can create the problems. For example, high and low referral rates to hospital in themselves tell us very little about the quality of care, yet are commonly used to suggest 'good' or 'poor' practice
12	Remove barriers that rob people of pride in workmanship	For health professionals, being valued is just as important a motivator as money. We all need to be stroked. In some practices the partners, as employers, overlook this fundamental point
13	Institute a vigorous programme of education and self-improvement	The 'learning practice'. The practice that takes on collective responsibility for the skills it needs, and makes it possible – and expects – people to achieve
14	Put everybody in the organization to work on the transformation	Quality in general practice is everybody's business

Berwick,[7] at the Harvard Community Health Plan, was the first to use the Deming principles on any scale in health care. He came up with nine factors necessary to make the improvement approach a success (Box 4.2).

Among all these principles and contributing factors to quality, Donabedian, Deming, Juran, Berwick and the Joint Commission on the Accreditation of Health Care Organizations (JCAHO) all emphasize the prime importance of leadership. Without effective leadership from the top, worthwhile quality initiatives cannot succeed. In general practice this means the partners, and it is of such importance that we devote a complete chapter to it (Chapter 8).

Box 4.2   BERWICK'S NINE SUCCESS FACTORS

1   Leaders in health care must take the lead in quality improvement.
2   Investment in quality improvement must be substantial.
3   Respect for the health care worker must be established.
4   The dialogue between patients and health professionals must be open and carefully maintained.
5   Modern technical, theoretically grounded tools for improving processes must be put into use in health care settings.
6   Health care institutions must 'organize for quality'.
7   Health care regulators must become more sensitive to the cost and relative ineffectiveness of relying on inspection to improve quality.
8   Professionals must take part in specifying preferred methods of care, but must avoid minimalist standards of care.
9   Individual physicians should commit themselves to continuous improvement.

THREE DISTINCT APPROACHES

The responsibility for implementing quality assuring programmes in the NHS has tended to rest with three main groups: the health professionals who provide care, the NHS managers who commission care and hold contracts for it and, most recently, patients as consumers. As we noted earlier, each group tends to have its own perspective on quality, yet, as we have just described, their separate identities are coming together under the unifying influence of total quality ideas and methods.

Nevertheless, it is helpful to see where each has come from, and is going to, so as to gain a clearer overall picture of where each links together, and where the gaps are.

Quality and the health professions

The professional bodies in health care make three main contributions to quality. These are through:

1   education and training
2   professional self-regulation, especially professional standards for licensure, the certification of competence after training and the accreditation of practices
3   clinical audit.

We deal with education and standards in Chapters 13–15. Suffice to say here that professional competence, to which both are directed, is an essential contributor to the quality of clinical decision making, and therefore to clinically effective care.

In this chapter we summarize the role of clinical audit.

Clinical audit: background

General practitioners became involved in clinical audit mainly through the Royal College of General Practitioners (RCGP). The launch of vocational training for general practice in the late 1960s was accompanied by the introduction of peer review and external standard setting in the newly emerging teaching practices. In the mid-1970s the College introduced practice activity analysis, an audit of the process of care in which practices could gain feedback about how they compared with others in relation to hospital referrals, patterns of visiting and so on. Soon afterwards the College launched its Quality Initiative.[8–10] The Quality Initiative invited College members to:

- specify the services they provide
- define their objectives for patient care
- assess their performance against these objectives and,
- where appropriate, change their clinical practice.

In 1986, the College published its Policy Statement on Quality in General Practice.[11] This proposed that clinical audit should become a basic method of quality assurance in general practice within ten years. It should extend to all practices, and should be integrated as an instrument of practice management as well as an aid to further education. These College-led activities were in parallel with, and helped to fuel, the growing number of clinical audits carried out by individual practitioners. The first major multipractice study of the effects of clinical standard setting in teaching practices got under way in the north of England at about the same time.[12]

The rest, as they say, is history. Mrs Thatcher's government, as part of the health reforms, proposed the introduction of medical audit throughout the NHS. In general practice the Medical Audit Advisory Groups (MAAGs) were established by the Department of Health (DoH)[13] to facilitate clinical audit in all practices. Audit within practice was stimulated alongside the growing number of inter-practice audits that MAAGs themselves carried out. Multidisciplinary audit soon came onto the agenda. And, most recently, there has been more focused attention on the audit of quality across the boundary between secondary and primary care.

Clinical audit: assessment

A recent review of the development of audit in primary care has shown that, since the MAAGs began, general practice audit has greatly increased in both quality and quantity.[14] More practices are doing audit, the range of practice team members involved has widened, the topics audited are more relevant, audit skills have improved and fear of audit has diminished. A recently published collation of evaluative reports on initiatives taken between 1991 and 1993 gives a fuller flavour of the work done both by individual practices and by MAAGs, for readers who want to dip into this area further.[15]

Nevertheless, there are gaps. Audit in general practice – unlike the hospital service – is a voluntary undertaking at present, and there seems little interest in making it a contractual commitment. There are still plenty of practices which have not entered the field. Moreover, within each practice, there would still seem to be a wide variation in the degree of interest amongst partners, with some keen to participate and others quite resistant. The concept of multidisciplinary audit rather than medical audit is still skin deep with very few examples in the published literature. And, even among practices that do engage in audit the audit cycle is too often incomplete, stopping at the level of the findings without proceeding to making necessary changes and checking on their implementation. A major stumbling block for many practices is still time, which is why it is a pity that much of the infrastructure money for supporting audit in primary care has gone on the MAAGs themselves rather than into the practices.

Data are still a major problem. As we said earlier, the data-based public health dimension of general practice is still relatively new, and so practices are not yet geared up by inclination, skill or technology to exploit their full potential for clinical audit or wider performance monitoring. Yet, data are the foundation of audit since audit is about describing, and about quantifying numerically. Good data provide the basis for the comparative analyses from which it is possible to see actual performance in relation to preset standards, and also to identify patterns that may provide the starting point for further enquiries.

In the modern practice, it makes little sense to think about the data requirements for clinical audit separate from the data requirements of the practice as a whole. Indeed, as practice information systems become more sophisticated and largely electronic, the use of data for audit purposes is but one aspect of what will become quite a comprehensive strategy for information management in the practice as a whole.

Clinical audit: a quality tool

This brings us to the use of audit as a tool for a practice to use for its own internal purposes, for its own development. In taking national clinical audit forwards, the main thrust has been directed to the use of audit for external comparison and review, which is only half the story. We think that its greatest potential lies in its value in internal performance monitoring.

Internal clinical audit has five functions in particular:

1 monitoring compliance with guidelines, both clinical and operational –
   are we doing what we said we would?
2 minimizing risk, by helping to reduce clinical and organizational error
3 as an aid to learning, by showing gaps in knowledge and skills
4 as a way of helping to bring about change by documenting the progress of
   change
5 in reducing frustration by showing why maddening things actually
   happen – regularly lost case notes for example.

Internal clinical audit may be carried out by a variety of methods (Box 4.3).

Box 4.3   INTERNAL AUDIT METHODS

- routine performance monitoring
- practice activity analysis
- survey and interviews
- direct observation
- significant event audit
- use of tracers

Significant event auditing is worth mentioning further here because experience since 1991 confirms the exceptional value of this method.[16-18] It is
economical in terms of time and money, a highly effective aid to learning, and
equally valuable as a simple way of recognizing error and showing how it
might be prevented in future. It can also be stimulating and enjoyable,
especially when there is good news to report and celebrate.

Significant event auditing is an adaptation of the *critical incident technique*
developed in the 1950s.[19] In operational terms it has evolved in general
practice through *random case analysis* used for teaching. Pringle *et al.*[16] propose
that the steps to be taken in the analysis of a significant event are as follows:

1 consider the events to be audited
2 collect the data on these events
3 hold a meeting to discuss the events. The meeting should cover some or
   all of the following points:

   - immediate management of the case
   - preventative care opportunities
   - follow-up of case
   - implications for the family/community
   - interface issues
   - team issues

- action to be taken, policy decisions to be made
- follow-up arrangements
4   documentation.

Significant event auditing can encompass the whole span of practice activity, both clinical and operational. Case Study 5, drawn from life, as are all the case

Case Study 5

Mr and Mrs Black, their son Kevin (aged five years) and daughter Tracey (aged one year), had originally registered with the practice two years previously. Mr Black had been a labourer then, but was now out of work. Mrs Black was a state enrolled nurse.

All the Blacks had active medical problems. Mr Black had chronic asthma, a condition for which he consulted Dr Adam regularly. Mrs Black had a long-standing history of undiagnosed, episodic abdominal pain, complicated by bouts of vomiting, especially in the evenings. She had seen Dr Baker regularly, but, despite extensive investigation, no firm diagnosis had been established. When bouts of vomiting occurred, the only intervention that gave reasonably prompt and symptomatic relief was intramuscular metaclopropamide. Kevin was subject to recurrent earache and had recently had grommets inserted. Tracey had recently been diagnosed as suffering from an allergy to cow's milk. When the children became ill, Mrs Black tended to take them to see the doctor most readily available.

One evening, Kevin had a further attack of earache and Dr Edwards visited him at home. Dr Edwards found no serious abnormality and advised no medication. Kevin appeared comfortable. The following day, Mr and Mrs Black took Kevin to hospital for a check-up on the grommets. They were told that one eardrum was inflamed, and that an antibiotic was indicated. Later that day, Mrs Black attended surgery with Tracey, when she saw Dr Collins. She asked Dr Collins how she could make a complaint about Dr Edwards who, she said, had failed to prescribe an antibiotic when the hospital doctor had said it was necessary. Dr Collins told Dr Edwards of the problem.

Dr Edwards was somewhat surprised by the complaint, because he had judged the child to be only slightly unwell and, as far as he could learn from Dr Baker, that was still the case. He decided to follow up the complaint with the parents, to see if he could find out what the problem really was, what seemed to have gone wrong and to try to restore relationships.

studies in this book, illustrates a typical situation later reviewed by this method of audit.[20]

Clinical audit: looking forward

In a recent report, the Clinical Audit Working Group of the Clinical Outcomes Group (COG) has made an up-to-date assessment, and put proposals before the DoH for consideration.[1] This report is important because it moves away from the concept of clinical audit as essentially a medical function, and as a function tied to education rather than to clinical practice itself. The report states that primary health care:

> will best be served by a strategy for health care which encourages, promotes, facilitates and where necessary requires each practice to have the capacity itself to assure the quality of its services to users, professional peers and purchasers or employers.

Clinical audit, in other words, should become an integral part of good practice management, so making it more likely that the audit cycle will be repeated until desired change has been implemented.

The report also makes the point that clinical audit 'should follow the patient'. All those health professionals who are engaged in the care of a patient within practice, and across the boundary in hospital care and in the social services, should ideally have their performance scrutinized in relation to their contribution to care. For example the audit of a patient with insulin-dependent diabetes would extend, using this principle, through the patient's general practitioner to the practice nurse who takes the diabetic follow-up clinic, and to the hospital when the patient attends there for further consultation or follow-up. Only in this way, it is argued, will real gaps be identified and remedied. The gaps are often at an interface, for example between general practitioner and practice nurse or between general practitioner and specialist.

Clinical audit, or rather the results of audit, are also more likely to have a bearing on the nature of the training and continuing education of doctors, nurses and other health professionals in future. To date, the linkage has been tenuous and the results therefore disappointing. The linkage between education and audit is likely to be sharpened even further as the drive for evidence-based practice and clinical effectiveness gathers momentum.

So, in the quite near future we are more likely to see a closer connection and inter-relationship between the three parameters on which health professionals lead on quality, that is clinical audit, the self-regulation of standards and training and education.

The managerial approach

The second general approach to quality is managerial, through commissioning and purchasing. The managerial approach to quality has assumed a new significance in the NHS since the health reforms. The basis is very simple, and is of course long established in the world outside the NHS. Commissioners of care set out their requirements, and these are likely to include indicators of quality and quality standards, as Case Study 6 shows.

Case Study 6

The Moores Health Centre is a fundholding general practice. It designated the length of the waiting list for outpatient appointments at the local district general hospital as a criterion of quality. In agreeing a contract with the hospital it attached the standards of performance it expected, expressing this in the number of days, weeks or months beyond which the patient should not have to wait, depending on the specialty.

This was so successful in terms of clarifying expectations and giving everyone, including the patients, something to gauge what was or was not acceptable that the practice then moved on to look at some aspects of technical performance by those with whom it held contracts. One involved the incidence of complications associated with hernia repairs.

Contracts for purchasing are simply formal expressions of agreements made between commissioners and providers of care. In the use of contracts illustrated by Case Study 6, early indicators of quality have tended to focus on factors such as access, convenience, communication with patients and patient satisfaction. Up to now the emphasis has been on the contracting itself. The evidence of effective monitoring, whereby the commissioner checks that standards agreed are in fact delivered, is limited.

Contracting for quality has other uses in health care. For example, most regional advisers in general practice now in effect place service contracts with trainers and their practices for a defined period of time, and within those contracts specify criteria and standards of teaching and care. Thus, for instance, most specify minimum standards for clinical records, and embody the use of clinical audit as a criterion of quality which they expect to be fulfilled. Postgraduate deans have been given the funds for young doctors in the preregistration year and are using the same principle with supervisory tutors.

Looking ahead, quality-based contracts are likely to become the basis of the relationship between the new health authorities and individual general practices. The shape of this is already to be seen in the guidance issued recently to fundholders setting out the commissioners' views of what they expect.[21] We cannot be far removed now from the kind of *rolling* practice contract that we discussed in Chapter 2.

Patient approaches

The third perspective is relatively underdeveloped, particularly in general practice. Nevertheless, the view that the consumer interest in quality should be reflected in all aspects is now gaining ground.[22]

The College of Health[23] has recently produced excellent guidelines for user involvement in the consumer audit of hospitals and general practices. These guidelines show how important it is to have a consumer input to assessing quality.

Pollitt,[24] in a series of thoughtful papers, has called for a rebalancing between the accountability to users and the accountability of professionals to themselves within the framework of self-regulation. Donabedian, in his Litchfield lecture,[25] has given an indication of the scope of this, and how it might be done. He assigned three principal roles to users of care, as follows:

1 as definers of quality, evaluating quality and providing information that allows others to evaluate quality
2 as targets of quality assurance, by which he referred to their role as partners or 'co-producers' of care
3 as reformers of care, emphasizing their role in improving health care systems.

Hopkins *et al.*[26] believe that the users of care must become far more involved in discussions about health care by contributing measurable outcomes of care that they see as relevant. Participation in research studies and contributions on the ways in which resources may be distributed are other options. The theme of user participation in the generation of new knowledge, which has an ultimate bearing on quality, was also reflected most recently by Richard Smith in a *BMJ* leader.[27]

In summary, there is little substantial evidence of engagement, especially within general practice, but this is a space to watch. The role of the patient as tax-payer and the impact of that in the debate about value for money is one that the profession will need to take on board.

QUALITY IN PRACTICE

With these approaches in mind we can now summarize the essential factors for achieving quality in tomorrow's general practice from the point of view of patients (Box 4.4).

Box 4.4   ASSURING QUALITY: PATIENT EXPECTATIONS

Patients expect general practice:

- to be patient-centred
- to seek high standards
- to assure good care
- to give value for money

This implies that the practice team has to deliver both professionally and in terms of the effective management of the practice. Boxes 4.5 and 4.6 summarize both functions.

Box 4.5   ASSURING QUALITY – PROFESSIONAL
              RESPONSIBILITIES

Professionals in general practice must:

- ensure their professional competence and performance
- behave ethically
- be outward looking
- be flexible and innovative

Box 4.6   ASSURING QUALITY – MANAGEMENT
              REQUIREMENTS

The management of a general practice must:

- promote leadership
- commit the practice to quality
- have clear aims and objectives
- encourage effective teamwork
- have good systems/data

To a great extent the arrangements and internal support that a practice develops to achieve these attributes are all under its direct control, and the next part of this book goes on to describe how this can be done. To underline this, in Box 4.7 we summarize the attributes of a quality assuring practice.

Box 4.7   THE QUALITY ASSURING PRACTICE

- appreciates the value of learning
- is ethically well-founded
- combines science and care
- requires explicit standards
- monitors its performance
- seeks to test itself against others

Clearly, the more a practice can manage itself effectively, and thus perform in a way that it both wants and is expected to do, the less the need there will be for that external direction and control that practitioners find so irksome. But no practice is an island. In Box 4.8 we summarize the main sources of external standards which will bear on a practice and influence the way in which it develops and performs. Registration and certification relate to professional standards of competence and performance, and are developed later in Chapter 14.

Box 4.8   ACHIEVING QUALITY (EXTERNAL STANDARDS)

- registration
- certification
- periodic recertification
- practice accreditation
- quality-based contracts

CONCLUSION

Quality in health care is a complex business. Practices need to have a grasp of the basic philosophies, approaches and methods for without these they will soon be lost. But with these they will find that they are able to develop their own approach, to build in their own values and standards, to manage in the style they find most helpful, and to chose a menu of methods for assuring and improving quality that they find particularly useful. Such self-sufficiency itself breeds self-confidence.

We have described the central role of criteria and standards in the identification and assessment of good quality care in this chapter. Clinical guidelines, which combine criteria and standards into statements of good clinical practice, are destined to become such key tools in clinical decision making and in quality assurance that we devote the next chapter to them.

REFERENCES

1   Clinical Outcomes Group (1995) *Clinical Audit in Primary Health Care.* London: DoH.

2   Royal College of General Practitioners (1994) *Quality and audit in general practice: meanings and definitions.* London: RCGP.

3   Irvine D H (1990) *Managing for Quality in General Practice.* London: King's Fund.

4   Lohr K N, Brook R H (1984) *Quality Assurance in Medicine: Experience in the Public Sector.* Santa Monica: Rand Corporation.

5   Ishikawa K (1985) *What is Total Quality Control?* New Jersey: Prentice-Hall.

6   Deming W E (1986) *Out of the Crisis.* Cambridge, Massachusetts: MIT.

7   Berwick D (1989) Continuous improvement as a sounding board in health care. *New England Journal of Medicine*; **1**: 53–6.

8   Royal College of General Practitioners (1978) Practice Activity Analysis 5: referrals to specialists. *JRCGP*; **28**: 251–2.

9   Royal College of General Practitioners (1978) Practice Activity Analysis 6: visiting profiles. *JRCGP*; **28**: 316–18.

10   Royal College of General Practitioners (1983) The quality initiative – summary of Council meeting. *JRCGP*; **33**: 523–4.

11   Royal College of General Practitioners (1994) *Quality in Practice.* Policy Statement No.2. London: RCGP.

12   Irvine D H, Russell I T, Hutchinson A *et al.* (1986) Educational development and evaluation in the Northern Region. In *In Pursuit of Quality* (eds Pendleton D, Schofield T, Marinker M). London: RCGP, pp. 146–67.

13   Department of Health (1990) *Medical Audit in the Family Practitioner Services.* Health Circular FP (90) 8. London: HMSO.

14 Humphreys C, Hughes J (1992) *Audit and Development in Primary Care. Medical Audit Services* 5. London: King's Fund.

15 Humpreys C, Berrow D (1993) *Medical Audit in Primary Care: a Collation of Evaluation Projects.* 1991–93. London: NHSE.

16 Pringle M, Bradley C, Carmichael C M *et al.* (1995) Significant event auditing: a study of the feasibility and potential of case-based auditing in primary medical care. *Occasional Paper 70.* London: RCGP.

17 Robinson L A, Stacy R, Spencer S A *et al.* (1995) Use of facilitated case discussion for significant event auditing. *British Medical Journal*; **311**: 315–18.

18 Beclin A, Spencer J A, Bhopal R S *et al.* (1992) Audited deaths in general practice: a pilot study of the critical incident technique. *Quality in Health Care*; **1**: 231–5.

19 Flanagan J C (1954) The critical incident technique. *Psychological Bulletin*; **51**: 327–58.

20 Irvine D H, Irvine S (1990) *Making Sense of Audit.* Oxford: Radcliffe Medical Press.

21 NHS Executive (1994) *Developing NHS purchasing and GP fundholding.* London: NHSE.

22 Joule N (1992) *User Involvement in Medical Audit.* London: The Greater London Association of Community Health Councils.

23 College of Health (1994) *Consumer Audit Guidelines.* London: College of Health.

24 Pollitt C (1993) The politics of medical quality: auditing doctors in the United Kingdom and the USA. *Health Services Management Research*; **6**: 24–34.

25 Donabedian A (1992) Quality assurance in health care: consumers' role. *Quality in Health Care*; **1**: 247–51.

26 Hopkins A, Gabbay J, Neuberger J (1994) Role of users of health care in achieving a quality service. *Quality in Health Care*; **3**: 203–9.

27 Smith R (1995) The rights of patients in research. *British Medical Journal*; **310**: 1277–8.

5

Clinical guidelines

It is virtually impossible in the absence of guidelines to know how to account for variability when we make clinical decisions

Robert H Brook (1989)[1]

We start by describing the general purposes and properties of guidelines, the means of developing them, ways in which they are currently disseminated to health professionals who may eventually use them in their clinical practice, and how they might be implemented effectively in general practice. We have emphasized implementation in particular because it is now generally recognized that securing consistent and sustained uptake is proving to be the most difficult step to negotiate successfully in bringing best evidence-based practice quickly to the bedside.

ATTRIBUTES OF CLINICAL GUIDELINES

Clinical guidelines are:

systematically developed statements to assist practitioner and patient decisions about appropriate health care for specific clinical circumstances.[2]

Thus, clinical guidelines:

should identify recommendations for the appropriate and cost effective management of clinical conditions or the appropriate use of clinical procedures with the principle aim of promoting good performance.[3]

Over the past ten years ideas have become much clearer about the general properties which desirable (that is effective) clinical guidelines should possess. The main attributes of clinical guidelines are set out in Box 5.1, together with an explanation of each.

Box 5.1   PROPERTIES OF EFFECTIVE GUIDELINES

Attribute	Explanation
Validity	Guidelines are valid if, when followed, they lead to the health gains and costs predicted for them
Reproducibility	Guidelines are reproducible if, given the same evidence and methods of guideline development, another guidelines group produces essentially the same recommendations
Reliability	Guidelines are reliable if, given the same clinical circumstances, another health professional interprets and applies them in essentially the same way
Representative development	Guidelines should be developed by a process that entails participation by key affected groups
Clinical applicability	Guidelines should apply to patient populations defined in accordance with scientific evidence for best clinical judgement
Clinical flexibility	Guidelines should identify exceptions to their recommendations and indicate how patient preferences are to be incorporated in decision making
Clarity	Guidelines must use unambiguous language, precise definitions, and user-friendly formats
Meticulous documentation	Guidelines must record participants involved, assumptions made, and evidence and methods used
Scheduled review	Guidelines must state when and how they are to be reviewed (under two separate circumstances – the identification or not of new scientific evidence or professional consensus)

Adapted by Grimshaw and Russell[4] from *Guidelines for Clinical Practice: from Development to Use,* © 1992 National Academy of Sciences. Courtesy of National Academy Press, Washington DC.

It is now generally recognized that much clinician time, energy and enthusiasm has been wasted in attempting to construct guidelines that do not perform in accordance with most of these criteria. Guidelines that are not rigorous may have the unwanted effect of endorsing practice of dubious value, or indeed of continuing to endorse practice which may be positively harmful to patients.

PURPOSE OF GUIDELINES

Field and Lohr[2] noted that clinical guidelines may be used for a variety of purposes. The most important they list are summarized below:

- assisting clinical decision making by patients and practitioners
- educating individuals or groups
- assessing and assuring the quality of care
- guiding the allocation of resources for health care (purchasing)
- reducing the risk of legal liability for negligent care.

It is essential, when considering the potential adoption of a clinical guideline, to clarify the possible uses to which it may be put at the outset, and make sure that those who are to use it agree and are comfortable with this. Nothing could be more disconcerting to the doctor or nurse than to find, for example, that a guideline introduced for the purpose of improving the consistency of clinical decision making was also to be used later, unannounced, as the basis for a formal appraisal. The necessity of securing agreement on use before implementation cannot be overemphasized.[5]

INTERNAL AND EXTERNAL GUIDELINES

Guidelines are of two types, internal and external. Internally generated guidelines are those formulated by the health professionals who will subsequently use them themselves and whose performance may be assessed against them. They may be constructed by an individual doctor or nurse, or agreed by members of a practice team. The advantages of internal guidelines are that they require practitioners to reconsider and reassess their current practice, a process which can be highly educational and therefore likely to improve competence. Moreover, the very process of working through current practice gives the participating practitioners a sense of ownership which, it is commonly held, is an essential precondition of sustained compliance.[6]

The problem with internal guidelines is that they are time-consuming to construct and may require a knowledge of technique that not every practitioner possesses. There is also evidence that objectivity is too often lacking because of the sheer time, effort and skill involved in reviewing the literature rigorously, and because of the understandable tendency for health professionals to glance over their shoulder, to see that what is being proposed is not too far removed from their current practice and therefore threatening. Internal guidelines may therefore vary widely in their content and rigour, and in themselves contribute to the very variations in the quality of care that they seek to limit.[1]

This explains the growing importance of external or national guidelines. It has now become clear that the effort, time, expertise and sheer financial cost of producing scientifically rigorous, evidence-based guidelines is beyond the means of local practitioners. Recognizing this, it has been proposed recently that national external guidelines, produced by authoritative bodies such as the medical royal colleges and specialist associations, should set out general principles of clinical practice for specific conditions.[7] Expert national guidelines may be produced by a variety of methods, including using peer groups, Delphi techniques and consensus conferences. Local (internal) guidelines would reflect the national guidelines but be adapted to specific resources and circumstances.

DISSEMINATION

The dissemination phase in the introduction of clinical guidelines, that is in taking the finished guideline to the clinicians, is very important. A wide range of techniques has been tried in the search for the most effective approach. For example, much weight is given to simplicity of presentation, to making the presentation user-friendly, and offering abstracts that the busy clinician can use with the evidence available as an appendix. Some methods of dissemination have relied on other media, such as the video-taped presentation, clinical conferences or incorporation in postgraduate education allowance (PGEA) peer group activities.

The phase of dissemination merges almost imperceptibly into the third and last phase, that of the active adoption and implementation by clinicians.

IMPLEMENTATION

The use of guidelines most commonly goes wrong at the stage of implementation. Yet this phase is so important that much effort is now being directed through research and development to try and reach a better understanding of the problem, and of the best ways of solving it. Effective implementation depends heavily on the attitudes and habits of individual practitioners in a subject and area where there is still much debate and un-certainty. In general practice the content of clinical guidelines today is seen generally as a matter about which individual clinicians should decide for themselves, rather than as a matter for the sort of corporate decision making by a partnership or practice team that we advocate and describe in the next part of the book.

Some practitioners see guidelines as valuable adjuncts to clinical decision making but are not prepared to have them used for managerial exercises in accountability or for purchasing. Others see them in neutral terms, simply as expressions of what they already do. Others positively reject clinical guidelines as an intrusion into their clinical freedom, claiming that practising medicine and nursing will be reduced to ticking boxes and following proto-cols; thus, clinical practice would be dominated by the *tyranny* of the clinical guideline. Still others are at a loss to know what clinical guidelines are, and what their potential for improving their practice is.

In the current literature on studies of implementation in general practice, there is virtually no mention of the importance of the partnership in enabling – or obstructing – the adoption of clinical guidelines, be they on prescribing, referral to hospital, attitudes to home visiting or indeed any aspect of the process of care. There is even less emphasis on how the practice team – embodying the non-medical members of practice – approaches collective decision making and, within that, the disciplines that a corporate practice or corporate team decides should be observed by individual members. Yet an understanding of what happens in this area is quite fundamental in seeking the way forward.

The importance of practice policy

Practices proposing to use guidelines will need to develop a general policy on their use, the key elements of which are shown in Box 5.2.

This kind of framework, if adopted by a practice as part of its general policy for its own further development, would substantially overcome the difficulties in implementation to which we have referred.

Such a policy would, of course, enable a practice to prioritize, and to secure and assign the resources of time and money needed to implement a strategy over a period of years. A practice may decide, for example, to take one or two clinical areas per year, to review these in detail with a view to introducing new or upgrading existing guidelines. New internal guidelines might be produced quite quickly. For example, one practice found the funds for a nurse practitioner and partner jointly to take two weeks' leave to generate internal clinical guidelines for the nurse practitioner to use in a variety of situations. A successful strategy will produce a balanced portfolio of guidelines for acute, chronic and preventive care, with generic protocols and standards on such generic matters as prescribing policy, clinical record keeping and clinical

Box 5.2 KEY ELEMENTS OF PRACTICE POLICY FOR
IMPLEMENTING CLINICAL GUIDELINES

Elements	Explanation
Awareness	Maintaining an active awareness of developments that could improve the effectiveness and efficiency of a practice's clinical services
Clear aims/objectives	Clear aims and objectives for care reflecting the practice's statement of purpose, and underpinned by its own well-defined core values and ethical standards
Agreement	Agreed purposes, role and utility of clinical guidelines and their uses in that particular practice
Mechanisms	Means of handling guideline development and implementation in specific cases
Educational policy	A general educational policy designed to help individual members of the practice team understand the issues in any particular clinical situation where guidelines are appropriate, and to close any gaps in knowledge and skill they may have
Audit	Used as a practical tool to help clarify a problem, reveal current practice and monitor criteria selected for review
Feedback	A general commitment to providing results to the corporate practice and to individual practitioners, for the purpose of reviewing practice – including compliance with clinical guidelines – and seeking improvement
Systematic review	A practice commitment to the systematic review of all results from guidelines implementation, with all relevant end users

---

Box 5.2: *continued*

Incentives/penalties	A collection of practice-based incentives and penalties designed to ensure compliance with an individual practice policy
General managerial arrangements	Designed to sustain compliance over a longer period of time, for example through regular random unannounced audit

---

audit. The strategy will be equally clear on areas where clinical guidelines are simply inappropriate. There are many such areas in general practice.

Implementation: the tasks of a practice guidelines implementation group

The most economical way of handling guidelines implementation is through the designation of one or two people within the practice to undertake the task of development. It is also helpful to identify the main responsibilities which such a group would have to carry. These are listed in Box 5.3.

Modern practices are beginning to see real benefit from the kind of team-work that includes delegation of tasks such as these to very small groups which can go away and get on with them (Chapter 10). Such groups need to report regularly to the partnership. Several practices have now appointed partners or senior non-medical members with designated responsibility for particular areas of practice activity, including quality assurance.

CONCLUSION

Within the next five years the use of clinical guidelines is likely to become widespread in general practice in the UK. Practices need to be independent minded about their use, for really sound guidelines are still a scarce commodity in general practice. Nevertheless, practices that have a positive outlook towards promoting clinically effective care for patients are likely to translate this commitment into action by making active use of clinical guidelines regularly and systematically in the ways outlined here, where they consider it appropriate to do so. Given a clear sense of direction, and a pace of implementation which matches the resources available, the judicious use

Box 5.3   KEY RESPONSIBILITIES FOR PRACTICE GUIDELINES
IMPLEMENTATION GROUP

Responsibilities	Comment
Ensure group expertise	Contains members who understand the clinical subject well and who are skilled in the techniques of guideline construction
Ensure group representativeness	Contains someone from each profession involved in the area of clinical care under discussion
Ensure patient input	Modern clinical guidelines are seen nowadays as incomplete without the patient's input
Clarify purpose(s)	There may be more than one purpose, such as use for decision making, quality assurance, etc.
Review and, if necessary, adapt national guidelines	To recommend to the practice whether any particular guideline should be adopted or modified for practice use
Identify obstacles to implementation and make recommendations to overcome	Mainly to do with people – attitudes, inappropriate knowledge or skills – or with general facilities and resources
Select and develop detailed implementation strategies	Such as the format best suited to potential users: *aides-mémoire* in clinical records; general reminders in doctors' and nurses' trays; periodic informal review groups to identify practical problems encountered, and so act as a spur to compliance
Select review criteria	If the purpose includes quality assurance, then the criteria in the guideline most suitable and appropriate for quality assurance review should be identified
Choice of audit methods	Advice to the partnership on the best methods (and the costs) of the audit methods and their costs needed for testing compliance
Analysis of results	For presentation to all involved in using guidelines

of clinical guidelines should be seen as an important new way of taking a practice along the quality road.

Guidelines are but one part of the cluster of new skills and tools required to aid clinical decision making and to assure quality. Ensuring successful use is essentially a function of practice management. In the next part of the book we develop the theme that an improved understanding of the fundamentals of quality management is central to developing both quality care and explicit standards of effectiveness.

REFERENCES

1   Brook R (1989) Practice guidelines and practising medicine: are they compatible? *Journal of the American Medical Association*; **262**: 3027–30.

2   Field M J, Lohr K N (1992) *Guidelines for Clinical Practice: from Development to Use*. Washington DC: National Academy Press.

3   Nuffield Institute for Health (1994) *Implementing Clinical Practice Guidelines: Can Guidelines be Used to Improve Practice?* Effective Health Care No. 8. Leeds: NIH.

4   Grimshaw J, Russell I (1993) Achieving health gain through clinical guidelines. I. Developing scientifically valid guidelines. *Quality in Health Care*; **2**: 243–8.

5   Royal College of General Practitioners (1995) *The Development and Implementation of Clinical Guidelines*. Report from General Practice No. 26. London: RCGP.

6   North of England Study of Standards and Performance in General Practice (1992) Medical audit in general practice. 1. Effects on doctors' clinical behaviour for common childhood conditions. *British Medical Journal*; **304**: 1480-4.

7   Clinical Resource and Audit Group (1993) *Clinical Guidelines: report of the working group*. Edinburgh: Scottish Home and Health Department.

Managing Quality

6

Managing practice

Management is too important to be left just to the managers

Glouberman and Mintzberg (1994)[1]

The previous chapters have made it clear that general practice needs to acquire a new approach to the management of patient care and clinical practice, particularly in its attempts to assure quality. Yet there are substantial obstacles to doctors' acceptance of the close and distinct relationship between clinical management and the management of people and organizations. To achieve assured quality care, it is necessary to overcome these obstacles.

WHAT IS MANAGEMENT?

The starting point is an understanding of what management is. Many people have described it. Drucker[2] said management is:

> the job of organising resources to achieve satisfactory performance, to produce an enterprise from material and human resources. Efficient management always involves a juggling act, facing different possible objectives and deciding the priority to be put on the multiple aims an organisation has.

Another view is that management is a process whereby

- purposes
- policies
- priorities
- procedures
- performance

are established, defined, reviewed, and modified.[3]

Whatever the definition, management is essentially an attitude of mind. It does not constitute a profession. There is no body of established and complex knowledge and skills, normally associated with professions, that can be acquired and that others can use. Despite this, *professional management* has become an enormously popular concept in the last few decades, and because of this hordes of people holding a masters in business administration (MBA) have descended on business. If this quasiprofessional view of management persists, it is unlikely that doctors will accept its central role in achieving clinical quality assurance. Clinicians will continue to use their knowledge and skills to commit resources in an uncontrolled way. This will create inevitable tensions in general practice as well as in hospitals.

Managers cannot be made in a classroom alone. As Mintzberg[4] says: 'the practice [of management] remains an art with surprisingly little scientific context'.

Effective management has to be rooted in a deep understanding of the organization being managed, especially in a complex organism such as a medical practice. That is not to say that people trained in a managerial classroom cannot exhibit such characteristics, only that their ability to do so has little to do with what went on in that classroom.

There has been much written about the functions of management, not always helpful. Nevertheless, some general principles stand out which apply in general practice. These are set out in Box 6.1.

Box 6.1 BASIC MANAGEMENT FUNCTIONS

- recognize the inevitability of change
- help the organization deal with uncertainty while moving towards overall goals
- introduce stability and clarity of direction in situations of rapid change or conflict
- underpin the professional activity
- ensure that the clinical process is supported by groups of appropriate and effectively functioning staff
- apply rules appropriately and consistently

Four kinds of skills are needed to fulfil these roles successfully, and these are set out in Box 6.2.

This part of the book discusses the key components of these skills and attributes, concentrating particularly on the human skills because management is essentially a human activity. Interpersonal competence is vital to its success. Any quality-based organization has to have a culture of consent and trust, with a management style based on persuasion and continual encouragement.[5]

> **Box 6.2**   MANAGEMENT SKILLS AND ATTRIBUTES
>
> - *human skills*, such as being a group leader, building and maintaining a team, and selecting staff
> - *technical skills* of decision making, priority setting, budgeting and planning, forecasting, establishing communications and information systems
> - *political skills*, such as understanding and using authority, wielding personal power and personal influence to advantage, creating the conditions for change, identifying organizational opportunities
> - *skills concerned with an ability to take an overview and see the enterprise as a whole*

DOCTORS AND MANAGEMENT

Doctors need to become more involved in management decisions and management processes, both to have an effective role in the Health Service, and to have an understanding of its management needs.[6] Griffiths[7] said: 'The nearer the management process gets to the patient, the more important it becomes for doctors to be looked upon as the natural managers'.

Some doctors, while initially perhaps being motivated by a sense of duty and the new demands of the Health Service, are actually now keen to improve their management skills to enable them to carry out these new roles. Some doctors find that accepting responsibility for new activities, such as effective decision making, prioritizing, managing people well, setting direction and planning ahead, represent a refreshing and stimulating challenge.

Case Study 7 illustrates the point.

It is still true, and particularly unfortunate, that the term 'management' deters many general practitioners today despite the illustration of its clinical value in Case Study 7. Time devoted to non-clinical activities is seen as less time for clinical work and family, which is why the priority given to organizational and management activity compared with both of these is understandably low. Management tends to be the activity that is done at the end of the day, or fitted in at lunchtime, or dumped on the most junior partner.

However, such random attention is not effective. Management, like medicine, needs firm commitment.[1] General practice needs to aim at recognizing that systems and institutions are like people in that they function best with steady, not just intermittent, care. Half-hearted management can be very damaging: good management requires more than a passing glance.

Case Study 7[8]

The partners in an urban general practice became fundholders because they believed that this would enable them to give good care while using their resources as effectively as possible.

In the early years, living within their drug budget posed no conflict within the consulting room, and the money saved was reinvested in other services for patients. However, in the fourth year, the budget allocated came much closer to real expenditure, overspending began to appear in the regular monthly figures, and the partners began to think they would end the year with a deficit.

This pressure made them all much more cost conscious, particularly in prescribing. They reacted by looking more closely at the detail of their expenditure and discussed the policies behind their clinical prescribing, focusing in particular areas that were most expensive. They scrutinized the clinical appropriateness of their actions and the quality of explanation given to individual patients. Sensitive issues began to emerge about, for example, the quality of some doctors' knowledge of prescribing and deficiencies in the practice's clinical audit arrangements. In these difficult situations the partners found that their ability to provide mutual support and to create a framework for improving the quality of clinical decision making became an essential, rather than a desirable, extra. In other words, the budgetary pressure had improved the quality of clinical decision making; it had not as yet reached a level that was thought to be harmful rather than beneficial to patients. If it did, the practice was clear that it would have to withdraw from the scheme.

In general practice the debate about doctors as managers is frequently confused. General practitioners are the owners of their businesses and most commonly hold the legal and the financial responsibility both for the practice as an organization and for its role in the community – the delivery of effective health care to the registered population. As such they have to take the key decisions on the direction the practice should develop and the policy framework for allocating resources – these are strategic responsibilities. How far the doctors involve themselves in the operational policies and activities such as budgeting, day-to-day resource allocation and information flows, depends on how far they are willing to devolve their centralized power base to others, a theme we take up in Chapter 12. The balance is crucial. Clinicians need to delegate to others to ensure that they release time to take key management decisions as well as time to carry out the clinical tasks that only *they* can. Any decision-making body within a practice, be it a clinical guideline group, a quality improvement group, or a building project group, must involve doctors in an active and informed way. Failure to do so will not achieve a satisfactory result for anybody, as demonstrated in Case Study 8.

Case Study 8

The members of a large urban practice decided that the pressures of clinical work were so great that they needed to employ a manager to take on the increasing burden of non-clinical, administrative and personnel problems. They were anxious to achieve this as quickly as possible, and, when one of the partners suggested an accountant golfing friend who was looking for a postretirement job, they leapt at the idea.

The accountant, John, had been a senior partner in a large firm, and was felt to have a great deal of business experience, as well as being able to look after the finances well. He had no clinical or health service background. The partners 'dumped' all the non-clinical activity on his desk, and he willingly took responsibility for it all. He was used to a disciplined and organized way of working, and had a rather autocratic style of staff management.

The partners were delighted. They received his reports at the weekly business meeting, and saw with pleasure that their accounts were looking healthier and in better order. They were pleased that he suggested cuts in both reception and senior nursing staff, and reduced staff costs generally. He introduced a performance appraisal system to increase 'productivity' by relating it to pay.

Unfortunately, there began to be many errors in the reception area, and a general loss of morale, reflected in increased sickness absence and an unhappy atmosphere. Eventually the senior nurse and senior receptionist complained of John's autocratic style and the increased workload, both of which they claimed were making it impossible for them to do their jobs. There seemed to be no advocate for them, or any way for the staff to communicate directly with the partners.

The partners were mortified and promised 'to do something'. When they spoke to John, he explained to them that the organization of the resources in the practice was his job, and that the staff had no right to go over his head. He would speak to them. The partners felt that, as they had appointed John to do precisely this, they had to leave him to get on with it. The following week both the senior nurse and the senior receptionist resigned, claiming constructive dismissal. It was the partners, of course, who were cited at the industrial tribunal, not John.

If the management tasks are being carried out by a non-clinician, especially a practice manager, then such a manager should not, and usually cannot, control the activities of the professionals at the operating core of the organization. These circumstances require a skilled and sensitive manager who can lead from the side, who can draw on the skills and leadership qualities of the medical and nursing staff and who can pull the decentralized clinical teams together to form an effective corporate whole. We discuss the role of the practice manager further in Chapter 12.

CLINICAL AND MANAGEMENT SKILLS

In carrying out their strategic management responsibilities and delegating effectively to others, general practitioners need to draw on and supplement the skills of the consultation in running the practice, and these interpersonal clinical skills should be used as the framework for managing the practice. Indeed, the clinical role of the general practitioner has many managerial components in its clinical activity. These include:[9]

- achieving goals through motivating others
- monitoring and developing the performance of juniors
- making complex long-term decisions
- organizing workload.

Moreover, general management, like clinical general practice, demands:

- the ability to relate apparently unconnected facts into a coherent pattern
- intuition
- continuity and on-going commitment
- diagnosis of problems
- consideration of options
- harnessing resources
- coordinating activity
- monitoring results
- persuading a third party.

Management is thus about analysis, persuasion, communication, delegation, authority and being a team player and a leader when necessary.

However, the analogy cannot and should not be taken too far. Clinical general practice has individual traits and characteristics that need to be borne in mind when comparing it with commercial or business organizations. It has no formal hierarchical control, and within the partnership there is no decision making by those with superior knowledge over those less skilled or experienced. As we have seen, the front-line workers (the clinicians) are also the owners of the business, carrying principal risk and liability. In a commercial business, a 'chief executive' may lack human or technical skills but still have conceptual and visioning skills. A subordinate can make up for these deficits and thus the chief executive may still be effective. In general practice, the chief executive equivalent is the group of partners (or, less commonly these days, the senior partner). Yet partners, because of the nature of their clinical work and their training, often do not have the confidence to delegate to somebody else the human and technical skills involved in, or to develop the conceptual skills needed for, running a large practice. The next chapters show how that situation can be remedied.

REFERENCES

1   Glouberman S, Mintzberg H (1994) *Managing the Care of Health and the Cure of Disease.* Paper presented to King's Fund Seminar.

2   Drucker P (1954) *The Practice of Management.* London: Heineman.

3   Irvine S, Huntingdon J (1991) *Management Appreciation – the Book.* London: RCGP.

4   Mintzberg H (1980) *The Nature of Managerial Work.* New York: Prentice Hall.

5   Prentice G (1990) Adapting management styles for the organisation of the future. *Personnel Management*; **6**: 58–62.

6   Berwick D M, Enthoven A, Bunker J P (1992) Quality management in the NHS: the doctor's role 1. *British Medical Journal*; **304**: 253–9.

7   Griffiths R (1983) *The NHS Management Inquiry.* London: HMSO.

8   Irvine D, Donaldson L. The doctor's dilemma. *British Medical Bulletin.* In press.

9   Tannenbaum R, Schmidt W H (1991) How to choose a leadership pattern. In *Business Classics: Fifteen Key Concepts for Managerial Success.* Boston, MA: Harvard Business Review.

7

Power as a tool of quality

A man's power means the readiness of other men to obey him

J S Mill[1]

WHAT IS THE EXERCISE OF POWER?

Management is the art of getting things done through influencing other people.[2] This is the 'power' which sets the culture and provides the context, meaning and corporateness for any organization, without which no quality of care can be assured. The concept of power is not one that doctors find easy. Indeed, the exercise of power can be an extremely ambiguous concept for many people. However, in all organizations there is a distribution of power, and it is important to understand that distribution in order to understand how the organization itself works. As Donaldson[3] says:

> Effective management hinges on knowledge of the sources of power in an organisation and how these might conflict and persuading people of the need for change and involving them in the process.

Therefore the exercise of power as a motivator is important and necessary for management, not in relation to dictatorial behaviour but because of the desire to be influential, a concern for influencing people. According to McClelland and Burnham:[4] 'A manager's need for power ought to be greater than his or her need to be liked.'

There are four types of power:

- position power
- resource power
- expert power
- personal power.

The first two, position power and resource power, both derive from the technical, statutory and/or legal appointment held by a manager or a leader. In the case of general practice this may be from the position of the doctor as owner and employer. Expert and personal power clearly both derive from the attributes of an individual leader. We explore each type of power in turn.

Position power

Position power is the main source of authority in society and in most organizations. It is exercised simply through everyone knowing each other's official position – the place in the pecking order. In today's society a superior position does not on its own entitle anyone to adopt an autocratic or directive leadership style. It does, however, allow some people to apply the rules and procedures agreed by everybody. For instance, it gives them the authority to call meetings, to initiate ideas, to appoint and select and, most importantly, to stop things that the power-holder does not like.

Position power is seen nowadays as not so much granting status as granting the right and responsibility to rearrange situations. Case Study 9 gives an example from general practice.

Case Study 9

John, the new senior partner in a seven-partner practice, announced at the first practice meeting after the retirement of the previous senior partner that he felt he should chair all practice meetings, even though the practice manager, June, had done so for the previous five years. John had not consulted anyone beforehand, but simply claimed it by virtue of his new position as senior partner.

The partners did not argue because they accepted that the senior partner role, while less influential than before, still carried weight and status. Anyway they did not want to offend him. The practice manager's views were not recorded.

Many managers and leaders in organizations tend to use the trappings of position power to emphasize their status. These can include badges or lack of badges, different uniforms, protected car parking, bigger offices, better furniture, separate eating and meeting facilities, better access to some facilities and so on. Unconsciously or consciously, many general practices have a number of the trappings of position power, which will include the use of first names, having a name on the door, making people wait, having tea and coffee made by others.

Case Study 10 shows how this can occur within the reception team.

Case Study 10

A large rural practice had a long-serving body of reception staff. This meant that even the 'junior' receptionist, Joan, had been with the practice for four years. Her family had left home, and she was now freer to do what she wanted with her life. Unfortunately, a precedent had been set that the holiday rota was decided on the basis of seniority. The 'junior' receptionist had therefore always received what was left, and Joan had for all four years had to take her holiday in August, the least popular month now that all the receptionists' children were independent.

Joan suggested that after four years order of seniority should no longer apply. However, the other receptionists were insistent that it should remain, and Joan continued to take her holiday in August.

Resource power

In many ways resource power is merely a subset of position power. This is particularly so when someone is in a position to stop or obstruct the development of aspirations of others, be it partners, nurses or the practice manager. If all of them are dependent, to whatever degree, for what they want – more staff, more equipment, more space, more facilities – then their dependency on the power-holder will make them more amenable to his/her influence than would otherwise be the case.

General practitioners as the owners of the practice have ultimate resource power. They give or withhold pay increases. They can improve or not improve the lot of the rest of the primary health care team through investment in the working environment. For instance, when a partner owns the premises in which the practice is located, he or she exercises resource power by virtue of the impact on the partnership of withdrawing that resource. Case Study 11 gives another example.

However, resource power is a two-way process. Whereas managers may be in a position to withhold tangible resources, they cannot carry out their job without the collaboration and effort of those who they manage. This is sometimes seen as negative power, namely the ability to stop things happening. Case Study 12 shows how this can happen.

Case Study 11

Dorothy Green had been the senior nurse of a large semiurban practice for 20 years. She ruled her team of five practice nurses with a rod of iron, but defended and supported them through thick and thin. She was feared and respected by the partners.

Dorothy retired in accordance with a practice policy of retirement at 60. The nurses felt bereft; not only had they lost their support and defender, but also they had not been trained by her to run a large nursing team or to negotiate with the partners. The partners decided that Dorothy's departure was an opportunity to save money, and instead of replacing her, or appointing one of the existing nurses as the senior nurse, they appointed two nursing auxiliaries. The nurses were asked to operate the department as a consensus team, and to delegate to the auxiliaries as much as they could. The auxiliaries were trained in phlebotomy, could take blood pressures, operate the ECG machine and apply minor dressings.

The nurses were very unhappy and threatened by the situation. They felt unable to complain or to discuss the matter with the partners, however, because they feared they would lose their jobs. They felt helpless.

The partners were quite unaware of the nurses' feelings, as they were more concerned with improving resource use, through both saving money and allowing the expensive, qualified nurses to concentrate on procedures that the auxiliaries could not perform, rather than carrying out minor, mundane activities such as taking blood.

Case Study 12

Linda was the practice manager of a five-partner urban practice. She had been the receptionist when the senior partner founded the practice as a single-handed general practitioner 25 years ago. As the practice grew, so Linda's responsibilities grew, until seven years ago she was designated practice manager. She was a patient of the senior partner, and was sister-in-law of another partner.

Case Study 12: *continued*

The practice had toyed with becoming first-wave fundholders, but Linda had been very unhappy at the idea. She felt they would bring in a 'whizz-kid' manager and that this would be a way of getting rid of her. The partners assured her that this was not so, but decided that they should back off the fundholding idea.

This rankled with the more junior partners however, and they began to see that every idea they put forward for change was met by resistance from Linda. Any effort to enforce a new idea, such as having name badges for staff or changing the surgery hours to suit the needs of patients, was negatively received by Linda. The staff were also negative because Linda modelled a negative approach, and anyway she was the conduit for all information from the partners. She became very upset if any partner dealt with staff direct.

The three junior partners decided that they would have to tackle the situation, particularly as they objected to having to ask Linda every time they wanted a new battery for their dictating machines. More seriously, they wanted to join a fundholding consortium and 'town rota' for out-of-hours care. The senior partner and next senior partner recognized the strength and logic of their position, but were concerned at the implications. None of the partners were involved in staffing matters, including paying wages, or with FHSA returns or the day-to-day finances of the practice. Linda's departure, or non-acquiescence, would mean a great deal of extra work for the partnership, as well as a great deal of unpleasantness and discomfort.

In the circumstances the partners decided they would have to wait for Linda's retirement to proceed with any of their ideas.

Expert power

General practitioners exercise a great deal of expert power – over patients, nursing colleagues and non-clinical members of the team. They have been the repository of all the expert power, but very frequently in a health service setting these days managers too are seen as having expert power and, as they become more competent, they increase their ability to exercise it. This to some extent explains the poor regard in which managers within the Health Service are held by doctors.

Case Study 13 gives an example of the exercise of expert power in general practice.

Case Study 13

In a first-wave fundholding practice, the senior partner, Dr Scott, and the fundholding manager, Bob Welsh, were the only two involved in the negotiation of contracts and the setting of budgets. There was a fundholding clerk, but she was excluded from the wider issues or the meetings with providers. Because none of the other partners was really interested in fundholding, and indeed a number had been luke-warm over the whole idea in the first place, none of them attempted to challenge the senior partner's stranglehold on knowledge.

Both Dr Scott and Bob Welsh were within two years of the practice's agreed retiring age, and therefore it was likely that they would retire together. The partnership attempted to raise the issue of passing on expertise and knowledge, but both kept saying that there was plenty of time. As the time passed, they began to suggest that they should continue on a consultancy basis after retirement, as no one else would be able to do it.

At this time the succeeding senior partner, Dr Leonard, decided that for good or ill he would have to get a grip on the issues involved, and therefore tried to get Dr Scott to share information with him. When this failed he began to talk to the FHSA and the Health Commission and other fundholding practices to acquire some degree of confidence in handling Dr Scott. He also encouraged the fundholding clerk to gain additional skills and knowledge, especially in monitoring the con-tracts, so that they began to operate as an alternative team, able to take over when the other two retired.

Personal power

Personal power is what someone brings personally to the task in hand. If your colleagues admire you and like the way you manage them, they will accept you as a leader and grant you real power. Such personal power is concerned with the totality of personal attributes – manner, style, charisma, presence, the ability to inspire – all very difficult to define. These attributes support the view that leaders are born and not made. In many partnerships the founding partner, the one who had the drive and vision to set the philosophy and style of the practice, retains a position of power by virtue of those attributes. Indeed, often when such a partner retires, the practice has difficulty in re-establishing a culture and philosophy that meets the new situation, rather than merely reflects that which has past. Case Study 14 makes this point.

Case Study 14

John Bull founded the Ford Practice in 1935, with Ben Smith and Ida Flower as partners. The practice had expanded, and by 1956 there were six partners. John had been a powerful dynamic figure, always the gentleman. He had been adored by his patients and the staff. He had been a caring and dedicated doctor who believed that the vocation of doctoring was the greatest gift. He had operated a totally patient-oriented practice, refusing to have an appointment system and never refusing to see a patient, however inappropriate the call. He had been a teacher of great distinction, and also carried out a great deal of research amongst his practice population.

The practice was a teaching practice, with a good reputation for rigorous research, excellent facilities for patients and staff, and lively forward-thinking partners. John had been very much the senior part-ner, not only by right of founding the practice and age, but because he had been an excellent chairman and good manager. He had spent much time ensuring that his partners were fully involved with, and took responsibility for, the various component parts of the practice's organ-ization. He had managed the organization directly through an excellent reception team and strong nursing force.

He had decided to retire in 1975. The practice was determined to maintain his high ideals and high-quality practice. Unfortunately, there was no leader in the partnership with any charisma who could take over: John's photo was over the reception area, and the practice name was changed in his honour.

Three years later the practice was in dire straits. Two more partners had retired, and some disastrous appointments had been made. The partnership was riven with dissent and disagreement, particularly over the workload. Nobody would challenge the basic philosophy of the practice and its applicability to the new partnership group. The man-agement of the practice was a disaster area, as the senior receptionist and senior nurse had both retired. The new practice nurse was of a different school and wanted to control patient demand rather more. The staff were leaderless, as the partners could not agree on the nature of the management they wanted.

It was only when the last partner who had worked with John Bull retired early in 1991 that the practice was able to find its new philosophy and way of working without the attendant guilt and sense of loss that had hitherto prevailed.

Those who might not instantly be recognized as born leaders can cope perfectly competently and efficiently as managers without personal power. The problem is that those who worry about not having such personal power can exercise too much of the other sorts of power. They can therefore become authoritarian, unfeeling, insensitive and dogmatic. Case Study 15 illustrates this.

Case Study 15

In a semiurban practice of six partners, the longest serving partner, Peter, was very unwilling to be the chair of the partnership. He did not want the responsibility, and did not feel skilled in any of the tasks his partners seemed to see him taking on.

As a result he took refuge in solitude, making decisions without consulting, telling rather than asking, setting the agendas of meetings without consent, and staying out of the staff common room where all the practice gathered. When challenged about this behaviour, he said that, as they had asked him to be the chair of the partnership, he felt he had many difficult decisions to make. Too close a relationship with staff and colleagues would make those decisions more difficult. He also felt he had to be the referee among his partners, two of whom had a stormy relationship. He felt he had to withdraw from them both in order to stay neutral.

He was seen to swing from remoteness and indecision, to authoritarian decisions and overfirm commitments on behalf of the partners. It was only when he started to make decisions that endangered the practice's income that the accountant, an outsider, spoke to some of the other partners. They realized that he was very unhappy in his role, and they were able to raise the matter in a partnership meeting, in relation to his poor health record in recent months. They decided to change the system and rotate the chair on an annual basis.

Nevertheless, managers who are motivated by a need for personal power are sometimes quite effective. They are able to create a sense of responsibility through their activities and creativity and above all a greater team spirit, but they are often not focused enough to be builders of the organization. Often their subordinates are loyal to them as individuals rather than to the institution they serve.

The increase in the numbers of women entering the profession is going to make a considerable difference. McClelland and Burnham[4] found that women thought of power as a resource to be used to influence outcomes and tended to focus on the competencies of people who work for them. Men in the study, on the other hand, tended to think of power more as an end in itself. They saw it as something they could use to react against or to take away from others in authority.

Men saw power as a way to supersede others in power; women rarely did.[4]

CONCLUSION

To conclude, the following sources of power as identified by Donaldson[3] are common:

- holding formal authority (e.g. the senior partner)
- controlling scarce resources (e.g. the senior secretary)
- having information (e.g. the senior receptionist)
- possessing special expertise (e.g. the asthma clinic nurse)
- displaying the ability to cope with uncertainty (e.g. the practice manager)
- commanding strong networks (e.g. the practice manager).

Effective understanding and use of these sources of power are the keys to good management, exemplified frequently in the ability to exercise leadership, the subject of our next chapter.

REFERENCES

1 Mill J S, essay on liberty.

2 Irvine S (1992) *Balancing Dreams and Discipline.* London: RCGP.

3 Donaldson L (1995) Conflict, power, negotiation. *British Medical Journal*; **10**: 104–7.

4 McClelland D C, Burnham D H (1976) Power is the great motivator. *Harvard Business Review*; **March/April**: 126–39.

8

Leadership

Don't let the round table fool you – wherever he sits, that's the head

Harvard Business News cartoon (1994)

If power, the ability to influence people, is at the heart of quality assurance, at some levels and in some circumstances leadership is the most important, urgent and dominant of the attributes of management. Every person with managerial responsibilities has to provide it to some degree, although not all are expected to be a John Harvey-Jones or a Mother Theresa.

WHAT IS A LEADER?

A leader has to be, in Tom Peters' terms:[1]

> a cheerleader, enthusiast, nurturer of champions, hero-finder, wanderer, dramatist, coach, facilitator, builder and carry out his leadership by means of passion, care, intensity, consistency, attention, drama, using implicit and explicit symbols.

It is the leader who has to see the enterprise as the whole, who can recognize how the various functions within the organization interact with one another and how changes in any part affect all the others. Leadership extends to visualizing the relationship of the individual business to the overall context, the community and the political, social and economic forces of the nation as a whole. To be a leader requires commitment, energy, a clear vision, a listening ear, an ability to create resources, an ability to set standards, an ability to recognize the importance of reward and the sensitivity to give feedback and to trust people.

Leaders need sensitivity to and awareness of their own attitudes, assumptions and beliefs as well as those of others. They will be skilful in communicating to others what they mean by their behaviour. Such leaders will create an atmosphere of approval and security whereby subordinates can express themselves without fear of censure or ridicule and in which they are encouraged to participate in the planning and implementation of those tasks that affect them directly. Above all, a leader has to have conceptual skills.

LEADERSHIP AND MANAGEMENT

The role of leadership is inevitably closely related to the role of management. Adair[2] has said that the leader is the person who is responsible for ensuring that the group has everything it needs to function effectively. If this is the case, then it is clearly true that leaders and managers are sometimes one and the same. It is certainly true that it is very difficult to be an effective manager without being a good leader. All managers, irrespective of their level of management, need to have leadership skills that will allow them to build a team out of individuals and to develop those individuals within that team in order to achieve the relevant tasks. This is just as essential for doctors within general practice as anyone else.

It is perhaps less true that you cannot be a good leader without being a good manager. A good leader may well have a second-in-command who is a good manager to carry out some of the more day-to-day management activities. However, the essential leadership responsibilities are, in Adair's 'action-centred' leadership model, broken into three inter-related areas:

1   achieving the task
2   building the team
3   developing the individuals.

A breakdown in one area will affect the others and prevent the practice from being run as effectively as it could. Box 8.1 gives a checklist.

Handy,[3] another management guru, defines a leader as someone who shapes and shares a vision which gives point to the work of others. The leader must describe and develop a vision of precisely why the organization exists, to what end and for whose benefit. In the light of this definition the leader must examine every single structure, process and approach to making decisions and all the activities that make up the organization and, if necessary, redesign them to ensure that they are geared to supporting this ideal.

GENERAL PRACTICE AND LEADERSHIP

We referred earlier (Chapter 6) to the traditional perspectives and skills of the doctors – those of observation, analysis, diagnosis, problem-solving and

---

Box 8.1   A CHECKLIST FOR LEADERSHIP

1   Achieving the task

- understand the long- and short-term objectives of the organization
- plan the strategy for achieving those objectives
- define and ensure provision of the resources needed
- ensure that each member of the team has clearly defined objectives or performance standards
- identify a resource group and individual training needs to close
  any gaps in ability to meet the objectives
- control and coordinate effort
- evaluate results and monitor progress towards objectives

2   Building the team

- explain the objectives of the organization and why they are
  necessary
- seek agreement on group objectives and standards
- maintain good communication and provide regular opportunities
  for team briefing and consultation
- offer feedback on good performance
- maintain team discipline and high morale

3   Developing the individual

- ensure that each individual has an appropriate job and
  understands it and recognizes its value to the organization
- identify and use each individual's special skills and knowledge
  and recognize that person's ambitions and needs
- provide a sense of personal achievement and ensure that all
  individuals feel that they are making a worthwhile contribution
- enable individuals to feel challenged by their job and ensure that
  capabilities are matched by responsibilities
- offer constructive criticism on performance and give support
  through an appropriate training and development plan
- give recognition for achievement and contribution

---

developing action plans. When they are applied to the broader picture of the organization as a whole, rather than to a specific patient, they serve as an effective framework on which to base management and understanding of leadership. Simpson[4] said:

> to be an effective leader requires an intimate understanding of the structures in the organisation; its anatomy (and understanding of the system); its physiology (the systems and processes); and the environment in which the organisation exists.

The Health Service in general needs leaders. The problem is that there are a number of relatively young people holding senior managerial posts, including that of partner in general practice, who have neither the maturity, interpersonal skills nor formal management training to lead a workforce of often strong-willed, frequently well-educated, professional staff. It is important therefore that leaders within the practice are not necessarily categorized by position power. They need to be individuals who understand and manage across the boundaries of all the dimensions of general practice. It is not the credentials but the knowledge and style of the individual, his or her bedside manner, that is important. Case Study 16 exemplifies this.

Case Study 16

In a small practice, the oldest partner was close to retirement and the three remaining partners were unhappy at the situation it left them in. The obvious next senior partner was part-time and she had neither the time nor the inclination to take the lead. The next partner was full-time, but very absorbed with clinical developments and not at all interested in the management or development of the practice. He very positively wanted to be led, and not lead.

This left the most junior partner, who was lively and dynamic. Although she had been with the partnership for only two years, she had shown herself to be clear-thinking and decisive. She got on well with the staff, both clinical and non-clinical, and seemed to be able to represent all views. She had the drive and determination of a leader. At the partnership meeting to discuss the next senior partner, they talked through the situation and were able to be frank about their own agendas. As a result, the junior partner was asked by the others to take the chair of the partnership.

General practitioners generally find the concept of leadership, or perhaps more importantly *followship*, a difficult one with which to identify. As we have seen, they work in a general culture that promotes individualism, autonomy and the idea of equality, to a level that is unusual in the 'managed' twentieth century. As a consequence they tend to find it particularly irksome and unacceptable to be seen openly exercising leadership qualities, and to relate to the leadership qualities in others.

Because of this cultural distaste for direct leadership, few general practitioners handle policy and strategic management comfortably. Indeed, in order to disguise the leadership demands of management, practices often have a very broad structure in which the areas of personal responsibility and accountability may be left deliberately vague. Partnership agreements nowadays are built on the basis of equality. However, practitioners have to recognize the tension between such a 'flat' management approach and the sort of structure needed to meet the demands of modern organizations and workforce, such as a sense of direction and purpose, and financial control.

Within this 'flat' approach it is possible to give the outward appearance of policy making. Partnership responsibility can be allocated and consensus policies can be identified, a framework for record keeping can be set up, clinical standards and operational policies can be developed, indicators for hospital referrals can be defined and levels of expenditure and methods of charging can be written. However, in the absence of leadership, agreement on such matters is frequently only skin deep, with no real commitment to the policies themselves or to their implementation. Case Study 17 gives one example of what can happen.

Case Study 17

A long-standing partnership of seven was transformed by the retirement of three partners within two years and the consequent arrival of three new young principals. The eldest of the original team, Geoff, was himself quite young, and an avowed democrat. He was the natural leader and 'ideas' man of the partnership. However, he was unhappy with the concept of leadership within a group practice, and believed that consensus was the way forward. His existing colleagues, Edward and Susan, overtly agreed with him, but the new partners, Elizabeth, Mary and Jim, were more concerned about the implications of such an approach.

The partners agreed that in the light of their heavy workload and the availability of suitable alternatives for patients, they would become like most practices and no longer offer intra-partum care. However, despite the agreement, two of the partners, Susan and Geoff, continued to offer this care, and frequently disrupted surgery by being called out. They were also often very tired after an all-night confinement. Their partners had to carry the additional workload.

When this issue of non-compliance with practice policy was raised at the practice meetings, there was chaos, as no one took control. They all paid lip service to the concept of agreed practices. Geoff exercised no leadership but insisted that consensus working was the right way for the practice to handle its decision-making.

His new partners pointed out the illogicality of his position and the unfairness of spending valuable time agreeing on a practice policy that partners then felt free to ignore. Because of his views on leadership, Geoff agreed with them! But he was not prepared to ensure that steps were taken to enforce partnership decisions.

As a result of this fundamental difference of approach, the partnership split within two years, with Elizabeth, Mary and Jim, the three newer partners, forming their own practice.

LEADERSHIP IN PRACTICE

Here are some statements taken from interviews carried out during visits to practices. They represent points of view about leadership taken from practice.

- Most problems are in the partnership's hands, and I leave them to carry the ball from there. I, as practice manager, serve merely as the catalyst, mirroring back the people's thoughts and feelings so they can better understand them.
- It's foolish to make decisions oneself on matters that affect people. I always talk things over with my staff but I make it clear to them that, as senior receptionist, I'm the one who has the final say.
- As senior partner, once I have decided on a course of action, I do my best to sell my ideas to my partners.
- As the practice manager, I am being paid to lead. If I let a lot of other people make the decisions I should be making, then I'm not worth my salt.
- I believe in getting things done. I can't waste time calling meetings. Someone has to call the shots around here and, as senior partner, I think it should be me.

These quotations show the problem of modern managers attempting to be democratic about their relations with other people, both partners and staff, but at the same time maintaining the necessary authority and control in the organization for which they are responsible. It is very difficult to devolve power, authority and budget responsibility while at the same time retaining a leadership position. The evidence is that the efficiency of highly directive leadership is very questionable. Increasingly attention is being paid to the problems of motivation and human relations. The continuum of leadership behaviour shown in Figure 8.1 demonstrates the modern situation.

Leadership today has to be tempered by the fact that employees resent being treated as subordinates. They may be highly critical of the practice and they expect to be consulted and to exert influence. People have tended to see the world as being divided into leaders and followers, but increasingly the concept of the members of the group has changed the way in which the leader can exercise leadership. Case Study 18 shows how this can operate.

In partnerships today there is frequently a reluctance to take the lead not only because of fear of being seen by one's peers to be putting oneself above others, but also because of anxiety about the amount of time, effort and energy involved. If those are over-riding considerations then perhaps the practice should look to others outside the partnership team who have the energy, time and commitment to create the leadership function that is so vital. As the case studies have shown, leadership can come from surprising quarters. It is sad that so many practices today are unable to make appropriate and timely decisions or deal with conflict because they have no

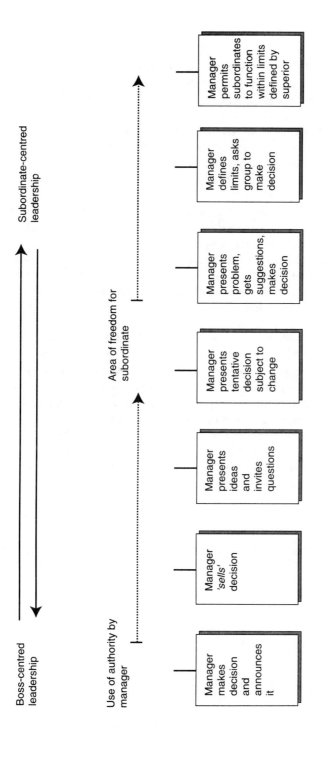

Figure 8.1 Continuum of leadership behaviour.[5]

Case Study 18

The staff of a large rural practice had a pay rise withheld in the fourth year of fundholding, as the practice income had fallen after the demise of health promotion clinics. Indeed, the nurses had not had a pay rise for three years, as it was recognized that they were well paid. The staff had been taken off the Whitley scale in the first year of fundholding. This had been done without consultation, but, as it was the only practice in the area, and most of the staff were patients, and the prospects looked rosy, no one complained.

Staff experienced an increase in workload and attributed the new building works that were being carried out to excess profit. They felt aggrieved that they had been told that they had to tighten their belts, when money appeared to be relatively freely available. The practice manager told them that he was devising a new pay structure that would not only give them a clear payscale, but would remove many of the pay anomalies that had inevitably crept in.

The staff were less than satisfied, particularly the nurses, and were unhappy at the prospect of another fundamental change to terms and conditions without apparent consultation. The nurses consulted their union, and the partners found themselves at the centre of a major and embarrassing dispute. They had assumed that the authority of the practice manager, backed by their own, would keep the staff in their place. They were wrong, and in due course, to avoid being taken to an industrial tribunal, they were forced to offer acceptable pay rises and appropriate reward systems. The attitude of the staff to the leadership of the practice was never the same.

apparent leader. They are unable to function as a coherent whole, a team. The next chapters begin to look at the issues surrounding teamwork.

REFERENCES

1   Peters T J, Waterman R H (1982) *In Search of Excellence*. New York: Harper & Row.

2   Adair J (1988) *Effective Leadership*. London: Pan Books.

3   Handy C (1994) *The Empty Raincoat*. London: Hutchinson.

4   Simpson J (1994) Doctors and management – why bother? *British Medical Journal*; **309**: 1505–8.

5   Tannenbaum R, Schmidt W H (1991) How to choose a leadership pattern. In *Business Classics: Fifteen Key Concepts for Managerial Succcess*. Boston, MA: Harvard Business Review.

9

Not being taken by surprise

'Now' said Pooh, 'What we need is a plan'

A A Milne

So far we have explored what management means for general practitioners, identified the power structure within the practice and looked at the role of leadership in general practice. We now turn to one of the most important functions of that leadership, and therefore management, that is to ensure that a practice is not taken by surprise by the sort of changes we have discussed in the opening chapters of this book.

WHY PLAN?

Not being taken by surprise is another way of describing *planning*, more particularly *strategic* planning. The purpose of strategic planning is to anticipate what may come round the corner. Some general practitioners take the view that the old well-established system of 'muddling through'[1] has served them well in the past, and they do not see the value of a more proactive approach. Indeed, they would argue that the events of the past few years have demonstrated that there is little point in planning ahead when external forces such as the government keep firing unexpected Exocets through the window!

However, there are very few total surprises in this world. The signs are always there to be spotted. For instance, in looking at any of the changes forecast in Chapters 1 and 2, such as those in information technology, evidence-based practice, salaried contracts, it is clear that the choice for any practice is either to read the signs and take control or to ignore them and be unprepared when they occur. Looking back, the signs leading up to an inevitable change in the general practice contract were clear to read several years before they happened. Only the final shape of the contract was unknown.

Similarly, the signs of a reorientation of the Health Service towards primary care have been developing steadily over the past ten years. They were evident to any who read widely, and could therefore appreciate the changing shape and direction of policy and the reasons for it.

Strategic thinking is also about ensuring that there is a proper map for the journey that the practice is about to undertake. What is the aim? Where does the practice want to go? What is the route that the practice is going to choose to get there? How will it know if it has reached its destination?

In our experience successful, and happy, general practices are those that have a strong, well-founded sense of direction. It is practices without that which are most often lacking in confidence, and therefore stressed and with sagging morale. This situation is not peculiar to general practice. Such a sense of direction marks out any successful organization. Not being taken by surprise therefore is about:

- reviewing the context in which the practice is operating
- determining where the practice wants to go
- setting the direction
- identifying the targets to meet to get there
- implementing the plans
- enabling the practice to monitor performance.

In other words, not being taken by surprise means taking control of the environment – shaping rather than being pushed. Case Study 19 looks at one example of this.

Case Study 19

Like many other practices, Meldon Surgery felt that the workload since the introduction of the new contract had doubled. The pressure on appointments was greater, more patients seemed to have more problems, the visiting list was longer and the paperwork more extensive. The seven partners were very unhappy at the stress they felt. They kept having emergency meetings to look at the appointments system and to devise new ways of dealing with the growing list of extras at the end of the heavy surgeries. They tried having a dedicated 'extras' doctor, they tried reserving additional slots at the end of the normal surgery, they tried leaving gaps through the morning to enable them to catch up – all the usual first-aid devices.

Nothing worked. They were like the crew of the *Titanic* moving the deckchairs around the deck while ignoring the iceberg under the ship. The practice manager produced data to show that the expected number of patient contacts in an average year exceeded the amount of doctor

Case Study 19: *continued*

time available by about 200 consultations a week. On this basis either more doctor time was needed or the partners needed to make better use of other facilities such as nurses or counsellors, or the patient demand had to be controlled by closing the list and improving patient education.

The partners were horrified at this. They each had a full day off a week, and an extra half-day if they were on call the night before, besides having seven weeks' holiday a year plus one week's study leave. There were two trainers with training sessions allocated, and two partners held clinical assistantships. The practice also looked after several private nursing homes and industrial appointments. All this meant a significant income above the national average, but also a significant limitation on clinical time.

The options put by the practice manager were clear, but to take control of their time and their lives, the partners had to face the real issues underlying the presenting problem of not enough appointments.

These real issues included:

- what standards of access should the practice set for itself and how many appointments are needed to meet those standards?
- what are the practice policies in relation to controlling patient demand?
- how much reduction in income is sustainable as a result of increased locums or taking another partner?
- what could be delegated to others in the practice, leaving doctors with what only doctors can do?
- what investment in patient education (including saying 'no' and drawing patients' attention to unnecessary calls and appointments) will the practice sustain?
- what should be done about doctors' appointments and professional interests outside the practice?
- should the partners' working week be lengthened?

The partners realized that they had to take control of their problems by making some fundamental decisions in these areas. They therefore set about defining these issues, and arguing out policies in these areas. They then defined the standards of performance they expected, and produced an audit plan to review the practice's attainment of these standards. They were then able to identify and choose options to resolve the real issues they revealed. The process, as can be imagined, was far from easy, because the discussion revealed underlying tensions between partners, as they all had their own expectations, aspirations and preferences.

Taking control has enormous advantages for the whole organization. These are summarized in Box 9.1.

Box 9.1   ADVANTAGES OF TAKING CONTROL THROUGH PLANNING

- improvement in patient care
- coordination and fulfilment of the aspirations of the partners
- ability to focus on future developments
- retention of control of the practice's future
- establishment of funding/resource requirements
- assessment of whether to opt for fundholding status
- ability to understand and use the advantages of the internal market
- establishment of a common sense of purpose among the staff
- staying in business
- success
- happiness

THE PROCESS OF PLANNING

Planning is probably the most important activity that a practice can carry out. Proper time should be given to it, time that is protected and not begrudged. It is also important to be clear who should be involved in the process. One view is that every member of the practice should be involved, that it should result from a collective discussion in which everybody has the freedom to express their own views. The outcome is, after all, going to be an end point for all staff, both attached and ancillary, and to provide a means of measuring performance and assuring quality.

The opposite view is that it is simply not practicable, or effective, for a team of between 25 and 40 to meet together in such a way. This view recognizes that, while it is vitally important that staff share in the planning in an appropriate way, relevant people should be brought into the planning process only as the need arises.

As the initial planning is concerned with overall direction and aims, those who have the most impact on the means of achieving such an object, and the most invested in reaching it, namely the owners, must be present at the initial stages. One of the most common, important and useful settings for such discussion is protected time out of the practice, often called an 'away day'.[2] This does not necessarily mean a trip to Madeira, but it can mean a day spent at a hotel or a partner's house, or more simply a meeting room in the practice can be set aside for the purpose. It may also be important to ensure informality. This is time out and not work; participants need to feel comfortable and relaxed. It is also important to think about whether or not an external facilitator will be helpful or whether the practice members feel sufficiently competent in understanding the processes involved and confident in their ability to understand all the issues that might arise to carry this out themselves.[3] Whatever the technique used, the idea is to end up with a defined and documented statement of objectives, strategies and action – the route to be travelled with its end point set clearly.

One thing has to be established at the outset, however. The development of the sort of relationship and culture within the partnership, let alone the practice, that will enable the emergence of a meaningful statement of purpose (*mission statement*) is a slow process. Thinking through is important to clarification and true understanding from which commitment flows. One 'away day' will not produce it. It is necessary therefore to plan the process over a period of time, to ensure that the energy and enthusiasm often generated on such occasions is sustained. Targets for achievements through what may be a fairly disjointed process can be helpful.

Often partners believe that the practice manager, if he or she is involved, can act as facilitator. It is certainly true that the practice manager may have a slightly detached or different view of the practice to that of the partners. However, this person has to continue living and working with everyone as an employee after the 'away day'. Therefore, the practice manager may feel inhibited about being as frank and directive as on occasions a facilitator will need to be. Such direction may be needed to move the discussion on, to keep to a timetable, to avoid a particularly sensitive issue, to move away from a dead end, to resolve an impasse. Case Study 20 shows what happened when a practice manager tried to facilitate within a partnership in a peculiarly sensitive situation.

DEVELOPING A PLAN

The statement of purpose

The first aim is to arrive at an agreed statement of purpose, often called a mission statement. Some scepticism is always expressed at the generalized nature of such statements. This shows some misunderstanding of the purpose. The idea is to reach the common point of agreement among a group of people. Sometimes such commonality is actually very bland, and may be a 'for motherhood and against sin' type of statement. Such statements, however, mean that there is always safe ground to which to return when the practice gets into areas where there is disagreement. Moreover, there is much value in the very process itself, if a practice takes it seriously, and is not

Case Study 20

In a four-partner partnership, the chair, Stewart, was a bully and a tyrant. He was thoroughly unpleasant to the staff, belittling them in reception in front of patients, shouting down the phone at them when interrupted and abusing them roundly if asked to do extras. In between being thoroughly offensive, he was charm personified! Most of the staff were long-serving and long-suffering. They believed him to be a good doctor, kind to his patients and the only partner with drive and initiative.

A new practice manager came on the scene and was horrified at what she perceived to be workplace harassment of both staff and the junior partners, two of whom were female job sharers. At the practice away day, she tried to raise this issue, by referring to the difficulties of privacy within the reception area. This was privacy for patients and for staff and doctors. Although she had spoken to all the other partners beforehand, when the issue arose, none of them attempted to help her or were as honest as they had been on a one-to-one basis. It was made clear that she was overstepping the mark by raising the point.

The issue was not debated, partly out of partner fear, but also because most felt that Stewart had given years of service to the practice and should be indulged. The practice manager felt bruised and let down, although clear that she was right and that the practice was in danger, because it was being exposed to avoidable risk of legal action for workplace harassment or sexual harassment.

simply producing what is often an anodyne statement for the FHSA. It can reflect deep thought by the individuals concerned as to how the statement lives for them, how will it translate into action and how much they will have to change attitudes or habits to make it work for the good of the practice and its patients. If it is worked through with serious intent then it will stretch and challenge the partners in a way that may be both rewarding and uncomfortable. It can be the means of producing either the lowest common denominator or, more likely and desirably, the highest common factor of agreement. It may also produce a level of honesty that needs careful handling – the subject of a separate note in Chapter 11.

Examples of statements of purpose drawn from very normal practices are listed below.

- To expand the range and quality of services provided and to improve the environment in which they are delivered in such a way that will meet patient's expectations, and that will be delivered by professionally satisfied practitioners and staff, while increasing the list size of a practice and being cost-effective.

- The practice undertakes to provide the best possible care for the patients, in a happy, safe and efficient environment. We will endeavour to meet the health needs of the practice population by fully utilizing the human and physical resources available to us.
- Our aim is to provide a high-quality service for the local population: to educate patients to take some responsibility for their own health and that of their families through lifestyle education; to enable patients to play a part in the treatment of any illness through clear communication and explanation; to facilitate appropriate access to all members of the practice team.

These may ignore some of the crucial issues of conflict within the practice, and be less than perfect in their expression and limited in their aspirations. They are, however, all products of hard and difficult discussion and compromise, and are sufficiently wide for everybody to agree that they are the overall end points. The greatest disagreements are likely to be concerned with the ways in which they are to be turned into reality.

Some people believe that statements of purpose or mission statements can turn out to be statements of the obvious or pious hopes. But a well-founded statement of purpose is not easy to articulate, especially if those involved intend to implement it, and it therefore carries commitment for them. Often quoted is the example of P & O in the 1980s when the company made an important discovery that it was no longer primarily a shipping line, but rather that it was in the leisure business. This made a substantial difference to the way in which it approached its customers and delivered its services. Similarly, the World Wildlife Fund, when it carried out this exercise, recognized that it was not a conservation organization but fundamentally a fund-raising organization.[4]

The SWOT analysis

A useful technique to ensure that a practice is not taken by surprise, and that there is executive planning, is to carry out a thorough analysis of what are the practice's good and less good points. Part of this process can be achieved by an external review by an experienced consultant. It may also be carried out internally, by conducting a so-called SWOT (strengths, weaknesses, opportunities, threats) analysis, looking at the practice's strengths, its weaker areas, the opportunities that are about to arise and any threats that it may have to face.

A convenient starting point for such an analysis is simply to list those external factors that the practice team members believe are affecting the future development of the practice for good or ill. Then to list the internal factors. We gave some examples in Chapters 1 and 2. Some more of each are included in Box 9.2.

Box 9.2   EXTERNAL AND INTERNAL FACTORS

External factors – some examples

- the implementation of the NHS and Community Care Act 1990
- the purchaser/provider split
- competition between providers
- GP fundholding
- commissioning
- medical audit
- greater patient orientation
- changes in the GP contract
- the introduction of financial budgets
- FHSA/RHA accountability
- reduced length of hospital stay
- day surgery
- community care

Internal factors – some examples

- indicative prescribing
- practice funds
- increased information requirements
- managerial changes
- new business or practice manager
- changes in clinical behaviour
- health promotion and prevention
- attitudinal changes

At its simplest, a SWOT analysis is looking at what will influence and contribute to the practice's development, what assets can be built on and what are the obstacles to be overcome.

Strengths may lie in the quality of people, services, reputation and image and perceived attitudes. Examples include:

- availability to patients
- young partners
- peer review
- female doctor
- branch surgery

- computers in consulting rooms
- daily partner meetings
- effective decision making
- low prescribing
- diagnostic skills
- time for patients.

Weaknesses can be inadequacies in the structure of the practice, the external perceptions, poor professional attitudes and so on. Examples include:

- high staff costs
- limited space
- poor standard of reception area
- insufficient training in the use of information technology
- high level of paperwork
- difficulty in implementing decisions
- the difficult partner
- lack of appropriate skills
- poor clinical records
- inappropriate prescribing.

Opportunities are those factors over which the organization has no control but which could offer benefits if properly tackled, such as we described in the early chapters of the book. These could include changes in legislation, public attitudes, scientific discoveries. Examples include:

- wider choice for patients with the development of a second surgery
- expanding practice population
- new teaching role
- involvement in commissioning.

Threats are events outside the control of the organization which could have a profound effect upon its operation. In general practice these may include, for example:

- changes in the GP contract
- political climate
- uncertainty
- competition for patients
- developing role of NHS trusts.

Once again, changing weaknesses into strengths and threats into opportunities requires the practice to take control. The 'ain't it awful' attitude does not make that which is awful any better, nor, more importantly, does it put anything in its place.

Aims and objectives

Not being taken by surprise means putting this SWOT analysis together with the overall aspirations of the practice. This should result in a clarification of the aims and objectives. An example, taken from a practice, is given in Box 9.3.

Box 9.3   AN EXAMPLE OF AIMS AND OBJECTIVES

To provide a high level of primary health care in line with government regulations, using our resources efficiently and effectively, being proactive in dealing with changing needs and requirements. To this end, we identify the following key areas:

1   understanding patients and their needs, and then ensuring that services and standards of care meet their requirements. In order to achieve this the following will be carried out:

- improved on-call arrangements
- a new appointment system
- new services, e.g. counselling service and continence clinic

2   effective planning of the use of all resources, including premises and equipment, and how they are to be financed:

- use all premises effectively, particularly the new extension
- carry out improvements to reception and increase the number of car parking spaces
- ensure that equipment is meeting patient and staff needs, including information technology and medical equipment

3   ensuring that all staff are fully trained, motivated and committed to the success of the practice and the care of patients:

- improving all communications in practice
- expanding the role of the practice manager
- fully integrating all attached staff and generating team spirit

4   ensuring that close liaison is maintained with the FHSA and other management bodies. Good communications in order to advise and seek support is vital in the current ever-changing environment.

THE VALUE OF STRATEGIC PLANNING

Strategy is the art of creating value. It provides the intellectual framework, conceptual models and governing ideas that allow an organization's managers to identify opportunities for bringing value to patients and for delivering that value at a cost-effective rate. It is a slow process, and effort and planning is needed to ensure that the momentum is sustained.

As Norman[5] says:

> In an economy founded on the logic of value, only two assets really matter: knowledge and the relationships of a company's competencies and its customers. Competencies are the technologies, specialised expertise, business processes and techniques that a company has accumulated over time and packaged in its offerings. The other key asset for any company is the established customer base.

Part of that art demands a new look at the relationship between the patient and the doctor. As we have seen earlier, general practice needs to recognize that a change is coming in the relationships between the patient and the general practitioners as the traditional provider of primary care.

Moreover, optimizing health care services in general practice means looking at new management techniques such as total quality management (TQM) and continuous quality improvement (CQI), to devise a new fit between the competencies of the practice and the competencies of the patient as customer. In the banking world the automatic telling system (ATS) and in the retail world companies such as IKEA have changed that relationship by engaging the customer very actively in their transactions. In general practice, the Smart card and the Internet may do the same for patients and doctor. The time to think about these future changes is now!

REFERENCES

1   College of General Practitioners (1972) *The Future General Practitioner.* London: BMA.

2   Irvine S (1992) *Balancing Dreams and Discipline.* London: RCGP.

3   Roberts G, Brown R (1993) Preparing for fundholding: the practice away-day. *Management in Practice,* issue 1.

4   Medley G (1990) Strategic planning. *Fund-raising Magazine;* September: 4–6.

5   Norman R (1993) From value chain to value constellation: designing interactive strategy. *Harvard Business Review;* July/August.

10

Teamworking

All together now

We have said a great deal so far about the ways in which practices should organize themselves to meet the new millennium. Many of those depend upon working together effectively. We look now at the myths and magic surrounding teamworking.

WHAT IS TEAMWORKING?

The current philosophy is that good general practice requires good teamwork to provide comprehensive primary health care. General practice tends to consist of both an overall team and a combination of special-purpose teams. In all of these, motivation, appropriate delegation and sensitive handling of people contribute to an understanding of what creates an effective team.

The words 'team' and 'group' are often confused, mainly because different people mean different things by each word. For doctors a collection of people working together towards a common end in a coherent manner is probably a group. For nurses it would be a team. The distinctions and definitions are often unhelpful and unnecessary, provided you define what you mean. For clarity throughout this chapter we use the term team.

We define the team as follows:

a collection of individuals or groups of individuals who adopt a common approach to agreed objectives and work in some sort of close geographical proximity.

Nowadays, of course, the issue of geographical proximity is less important. The impact of remote technology on teamworking is beginning to be discussed. Handy[1] has described organizations that are now more like a con-dominium, that is an association of residents gathered together for mutual convenience. The age of the organization as we know it may be coming to an end, and therefore the role of teamwork may be changing rapidly. Organizations will continue to organize themselves and their activities but they may not need to do it through a directly employed labour force. In a people-oriented business, such as general practice, the impact is likely to be great because of the dependency on part-time married women and the shifting nature of much of the work, be it clinical or clerical.

The view expressed in this chapter is that teams and teamworking are organizational and management tools. Bearing in mind the relationship between clinical management and organizational management which we have emphasized so far, the experience of most doctors will be of working in clinical teams. These, when they are multidisciplinary, tend to have as many difficulties and tensions as organizational teams.

WHY TEAMBUILD?

Teams and teambuilding are needed to ensure consistency between individual members of the practice and the delivery of the practice aspirations. The overall objectives of health care may well be shared within a practice, but the methods by which such objectives can be achieved are likely to stimulate considerable differences of view among those who contribute to their achievement. Furthermore, the tensions between administrative and financial efficiency and clinical efficacy can create significant challenges for the multidisciplinary team. There is a risk that rivalry and a polarization of views may become a major obstacle to the full development of teamwork in general practice. An environment that creates and encourages participation can be used to turn this tension and stimulus into a strength to handle the range of activities offered in the practice and may help people work together in a significant way. Case Study 21 illustrates this point.

At the same time differing perspectives, personal goals and views about the clinical directions need to be addressed. To achieve this, members of each team need a shared understanding of one another's potential contribution and actual function. Team members need to understand what their role contributes to the roles of others. Patients coming into a practice base their total experience on the basis of the ease with which they get appointments, get through on the telephone, how kind the nurse is and so on. Each person with whom the patient comes into contact is contributing to the image of the practice team.

Moreover, as we have discussed, modern management is beginning to shed the old hierarchical structure and is learning to value each member of the team's contribution. In this way, everybody can feel responsible for the performance of the whole team and not operate alone. Team cohesion is

Case Study 21

A practice in the heart of Inner London consisted of seven partners, four practice nurses, two counsellors, two interpreters, three attached social workers, a visiting nutritionist, a practice manager, two assistant practice managers, a senior receptionist and full receptionist team, three secretaries, a computer manager and operator, and all the attached usual nursing staff. It had become obvious to the partners and practice manager that true multidiscipinary teamwork was the only way to ensure that such a large organization worked to give job satisfaction for all. The only alternative would have been autocracy, and that was not acceptable to the partners, even if the orderly practice manager had a sneaking liking for it! Although the day-to-day maintenance of the practice was the job of the practice manager and her assistants, the partners were clear that it was vital to have everybody on board when it was looking at new developments. These included enlarging its premises; trying to attract hospital consultants to run clinics at the surgery; the nurse practitioner role; developing staff appraisal and job development systems; introducing new clinical guidelines. There were many more ideas.

To try to achieve an agreed priority listing, the partners called a staff meeting in protected time, that is they shut the surgery for a half-day after giving the patients due notice and employed a locum receptionist (a previous receptionist who had left after having a baby) and a locum doctor to take emergency calls. At the meeting everyone had their say and a list of priorities was produced, to which everyone subscribed.

Staff were then asked to sign up to a series of working parties set up to design and implement the top priorities. This was the extension to the building, and the working party for that attracted 20! At the first meeting of this team, several people said that it was too unwieldy. The senior receptionist was the most vocal, and suggested that there were so many elements to the new building that they should divide the tasks up according to skill and interest. They should have a series of teams – one on the finance, one on the space needs, one on the income generation possibilities, one on the patient involvement, one on the interior design and fittings. Each of these teams elected a representative to sit on a management team of five or six which coordinated the scheme and liaised most closely with the architect. The teams were diverse in terms of profession and background, and everyone tended to forget who was what in their professional lives when they were

Case Study 21: *continued*

working in their small team. Most teams met out of hours, often at people's homes, and meetings were often followed by a meal.

There were no instances of conflict, design versus finance for instance, and at the successful completion of the project everyone agreed that it had been an excellent example of using teambuilding to complete a project effectively. More importantly, hidden talents were revealed or created, not necessarily related to an individual's professional skill.

The practice used the same approach for devising local clinical guidelines and operational protocols. The receptionists turned out to have some very stimulating ideas on how to make sure that clinics worked effectively and in working out protocols for obtaining emergency access to doctors.

greater when individual members view their fate as depending on the functioning of the team as a whole. In the same way, a manager who helps individuals achieve their personal fulfilment is consolidating team development.

HOW DO PEOPLE WORK TOGETHER?

There are three ways that people come together.

1 Managers tend to put people together to get work done in a project team. This might be a quality improvement group or the partnership might form itself into a board to manage the overall practice.
2 People form themselves naturally into teams to protect their interests. The most obvious of these are trade unions or professional associations, a young principals group or the local practice managers' forum or the practice nurse team.
3 People satisfy their basic human need for belonging by being members of informal groups or sports teams or clubs. This might be a ten-pin bowling practice team or a receptionists' cinema club or merely a group that goes out for dinner quite often.

Teams work through the personalities and different styles of individual members. Psychometric testing can be used to explore the dynamics of these teams. Honey and Mumford[2] have classified people as :

- *activists*, who take decisions quickly but perhaps do not consider all the ramifications and tend to be impatient towards team members who work more slowly

- *reflectors*, who debate and consider decisions carefully, which may lead to quality of thought but obstruct process
- *theorists*, who offer systematic and logical arguments and can therefore usefully dispel complacency but can be diffident in reaching a sensible consensus
- *pragmatists*, who can be relied on to identify problems and their solutions but may be driven down rigid channels rather than theorizing over all the options.

In partnerships particularly it is important to know what sort of individuals and personalities are present. If there is a distorting preponderance of one style among individuals in a team then there will be difficulty in creating an effective balance. Case Study 22 gives an example.

Case Study 22

Ian was the driving force of a partnership of five. He attracted lively new partners, in particular Graham, who was another dynamic personality. Ian had many outside interests. He was active in the RCGP, and was nationally involved with audit and education. As a result, the practice was often in the vanguard of developments, and frequently acted as a pilot for experimental schemes. Graham was developing the same interests, and the other partners were very happy to reflect in their glory and enjoy the challenges Ian brought, although they were less enthusiastic about the extra work it all involved.

Graham decided at 40 to change his career and go into full-time academic general practice. This was a great blow to Ian, who had seen him as his successor in the driving seat. The other partners were less unhappy. They saw replacing Graham as an opportunity to bring in another quieter and more reflective partner, and create what they saw as a period of stability. They outvoted Ian and selected a very quiet and conscientious mature partner, George.

Ian retired five years later, and the partners found themselves with no *activist* or much in the way of a *pragmatist*. They appointed another *reflector*, without considering where the drive and energy for the practice to move forward was going to come from. As a result, the practice stagnated and the partners and staff became bored and frustrated.

Similarly Belbin[3] identified four broad types of personalities, which he described as:

1 leaders
2 administrators
3 drivers
4 ideas people.

Within these headings he identified eight groupings of individual behaviour that both positively and negatively affect teamwork. These are as follows:

1 the leaders – those able to coordinate a group (chairs) and those able to shape the views of the group (shapers)
2 the administrators – teamworkers and those able to evaluate and monitor the performance of the group (monitor evaluators)
3 the drivers – those providing the bedrock of workers (company workers) and those able to work through issues and projects to the end (completer finishers)
4 ideas people – those able to investigate the best way of using resources (resource investigators) and those initiating new ideas (plants).

Using these scales it is possible, as done by Honey and Mumford, to map broadly the styles and personalities in any given team and to indicate the team strengths and weaknesses in different areas of contribution. For instance, too much plant and not enough company worker may mean that you are in a team that is strong on ideas but weak on execution. Similarly, too much monitor evaluator and not enough shaper may mean you have a team that lacks ideas. A balance of styles is desirable. But it is equally desirable, if not essential to effective working, to have leadership skills within the group. Chapter 8 dwelt in more detail on the attributes of a leader, but specifically in this instance one would be looking for the ability to master the subject under discussion and skills in handling group dynamics.

DEVELOPING A TEAM

The manager's task is to reduce conflict among so many different team types.[4] There are four usually recognized stages of team development, explicitly put by Handy[5] as forming, storming, norming and performing. It is worth being aware of these.

Forming

At this stage the team is not yet a coherent whole but a set of individuals who tend to talk about the purpose of the team, its definition, its title, its composition, its leadership, its lifespan. At this stage, too, each individual tends to want to establish his or her personal identity within the team and make some individual impression. In practice, this might be, for example, the early stages of deciding on a taskforce to coordinate the development of the clinical audit of chronic disease, where the ideas are flowing freely on what to audit but there is as yet no clear order of process, leader or timescale.

Storming

Most teams go through a conflict stage during which the original enthusiasm and apparent agreement on purpose, leadership and other roles is challenged and re-established. At this stage many personal agendas are revealed and a certain amount of interpersonal hostility can be generated. This can lead to a more realistic setting of objectives, procedures and processes. For example, there are stages in the taskforce meetings when the nurses and the doctors disagree over what data should be collected, how best to show good practice by one professional group at the expense of another and who should do the work.

Norming

The team needs to establish its style of operation and practices, such as when and how it should work, how it should take decisions and what type of behaviour, what level of work and what degree of openness, trust and confidence are appropriate. At this stage there will be much tentative experimentation by individuals within the practice to measure the tenor of the team and to assess the appropriate level of commitment.

Performing

It is only when the three previous stages have been successfully completed that any team reaches full maturity and is able to be fully and sensibly productive. Some kind of performance will be achieved at all stages of development, but it is likely to be impeded by the other processes of growth and by individual agendas in the example given. It is at this stage that the taskforce becomes a team and is able to agree its aims and processes.

WHAT IS AN EFFECTIVE TEAM?

It is certainly easy to identify what are the indications of *ineffective* teamworking:

- performing below expected standards
- people blaming others
- forming cliques or unexpected liaisons
- displays of aggressive or destructive behaviour
- a loss of interest in the team's activity
- passing on problems for others to deal with.

Some of the factors inherent in an ineffective team are listed below:

- too large
- member characteristics
- too many individual agendas
- impossible nature of the task
- lack of or overwhelming importance of the task
- lack of clarity of the task description or lack of shared objectives
- weak position of the leader
- uncomfortable and unsuitable physical location
- insufficient time
- lack of motivation of individuals
- lack of teambuilding skill.

By default, looking at these in more detail reveals some of the factors involved in effective teamworking.

Size

Clearly, the larger the team the greater the pool of talent, skills and knowledge but also the less chance of individual participation. It is a trade-off. Practical experience indicates that a size of between five and seven is the optimum. If the team needs to be larger, then the role of the leader or chair will be that much more important in dealing with the participants, their influence and potential conflict.

Member characteristics

Awareness of the sort of roles played by people as identified by Honey and Mumford or by Belbin is important, particularly when there is a predominance of any one type.

Individual agendas

It is patently obvious that, if all members of a team have the same objectives, the group will tend to be that much more effective. But it is also true that, in most teams, most people have hidden agendas. These will include:

- the protection of personal interests
- the need to impress colleagues
- the need to score off somebody else
- the need to make an alliance with somebody else
- the need to cover up errors.

The interesting thing about hidden agendas is that they can disappear when there is a common crisis or enemy, such as a flu epidemic. This can be dangerous as the team can become too cohesive and hidden agendas may be buried. This would actually tend to lead to teams being blind to all the ramifications of a particular decision.

The nature of the task

The nature of the task will clearly have an impact on the nature of the team. If it is purely for information dissemination then there will be quite a different impact than if it is a problem-solving team, or, as in partnership, a management team. Different teams need different identities fixed by title, place and time, and the nature of the task or tasks for the team needs to be clearly identified to ensure the effective working of the team. In the same way, the more important the task to the individual the more committed the member will be to the team and the less concerned about his or her own objectives. Similarly, the organization is likely to pay more attention to the team's performance if it is a team that is fairly central to the overall purpose of the organization.

In general, therefore, the more important the task, the more the organization can demand of a particular team. Conversely, the organization is more likely to want to control the team and therefore demotivate it. If teams or committees are convened or constructed for an inappropriate task or with impossible constraints, if they are badly led or have ineffective procedures, if they have the wrong people, too many people, too little power or meet too infrequently, if in short any one of part of the requirements is out of place, frustration will set in and anarchy will be created. The result will be either an activation of negative power or a badly attended, non-effective team, wasting people's time and space.

IS A TEAM ALWAYS NECESSARY?

It is important to add just a word of warning. Teams there must be. Individuals must be coordinated and their skills and abilities meshed and merged, but the emphasis on teamworking should not remove the need to assess very carefully when a team is needed. Frequently the value of a full-blooded team operation can be devalued by worshipping at the shrine of teambuilding. Rather we should use ad hoc cooperative groups or networks or even recognize where an activity or issue merely needs good communication between individuals. The levels of working can be defined from dealing with simple issues or puzzles to more complex puzzles to major problems. Simple, often technical, issues which arise inside a group or in relation to one member's technical function can merely require individuals literally to mind their own business. The question is do we need a team to address this particular problem. Case Study 23 illustrates this point.

Case Study 23

In a semi-rural practice with three partners and a practice manager, there were continuing complaints about the inefficient telephone system. The practice manager, Jo, brought it to the partners' attention, and the senior partner, Malcolm, suggested that Jo and one of the other partners should get together with a receptionist and a nurse to form a team to investigate and make recommendations on a new system. Jo suggested that, as she had been involved in the selection of a telephone system before, she should do the research, and seek the views of others as necessary. The partners agreed, and Jo produced a range of options for discussion among the staff and the partners. They had demonstrations of three, and made a selection. As a result of not setting up a team, the practice reckoned that they had saved some three months in implementation.

In more complex situations it will of course be necessary for the management team to carry out most of the problem-solving work, particularly where there are questions that no one member of the team can handle alone. Choosing a new computer system is one such issue, involving as it does a range of skills, as Case Study 24 shows.

Case Study 24

The same practice decided to change its computer system. The partners talked to Jo, the practice manager, about whether she felt able to do the preliminary searching without help. Jo suggested that, unlike the telephone system, of which she had expertise and which involved a relatively small amount of money, the computer system was a vital part of the practice's working for every member and would represent a large financial investment. The practice therefore set up a multidisciplinary team consisting of one partner, Jo, the senior practice nurse, the secretary and senior receptionist. The team researched together and separately and, when they had agreed their options, they presented them to the whole practice. They had been sufficiently representative and carried out sufficient consultation along the way for it to be agreed without dissent.

Teamworking becomes even more vital and valuable when management issues become very complex and complicated. Problems that have considerable consequences, particularly major resource implications, are clear examples of this and will usually fall to the partnership team. The most obvious of these is the decision of a partnership to apply to become a fundholding practice. Case Study 25 continues with the same practice.

Case Study 25

When one of the partners raised the issue of fundholding at a practice meeting, Jo, the practice manager, offered to research the issues involved with the accountant. The partners felt that, as the issue was so vital to the strategic direction of the practice, they as the partnership team had to investigate the matter personally. They planned a series of visits to neighbouring fundholding practices and had meetings with the FHSA and the accountant. When they felt they had enough information to make a decision in principle, they had some time out of the practice as a team to thrash out the philosophical and professional issues for them as clinicians and as partners of the firm. Only after they had resolved the issues in their own minds did they invite additional members of the practice, including of course the practice manager, to give their views and participate in discussion on the practicalities of implementation.

So the most discriminating questions are:

- does any of your work as a management group require you to be a team?
- do you have a major problem to face or is it merely a puzzle to be sorted out by a technical or local expert group or by individual members themselves?

If these questions are answered thoughtfully, then teamwork will be used sparingly, limited to those situations that could not be handled by an individual or one or two people appropriately. Teamwork used in this way makes the most effective use of one's time and the skills available.

REFERENCES

1   Handy C (1989) *The Age of Unreason*. London: Business Books.

2   Honey P, Mumford A (1986) *A Manual of Learning Styles*. Maidenhead, Berks: Honey.

3   Belbin M (1981) *Management Teams – Why they Succeed and Fail*. London: Heineman.

4   Kramer H E (1975) The philosophical foundations of management rediscovered. *Management International Review*; **15**: 2–3.

5   Handy C (1994) *The Empty Raincoat*. London: Hutchinson.

11

The partnership team

By uniting we stand, by dividing we fall

John Dickinson (1732–1808)

In our experience, the most difficult part of the business of general practice is managing the partner team. The central role that this team plays in the effective delivery of assured quality justifies a chapter on its own, a chapter sprinkled with more case studies drawn from life.

Doctors are not by culture or tradition strong team players. The nature of their profession, with each doctor carrying ultimately named responsibility for individual patients, dictates an organization of single players, albeit supported by their own team of juniors, especially in hospital. This means that many doctors gain little experience of working as equal players in teams throughout their training. The modelling that they receive as registrars may not be helpful.

Nevertheless, most general practitioners choose to operate within a partnership, which is a very strong and formal arrangement. Most partnerships operate primarily at the legal and constitutional level, with little thought for the implications for behaviour, management or interpersonal responsibilities. The greatest challenge is to bring practitioners together regularly, so they can agree and commit themselves to objectives and standards of care, together with any changes in practice policy and personal behaviour deemed necessary. Case Study 26 reflects this.

One of the commonest major problems in handling this kind of situation is the unwillingness of partnerships to handle confrontation and conflict within their ranks. Many partners are concerned primarily with retaining harmony. This is understandable given that their biggest fear is the disruption of the partnership. Lack of honesty and overt agendas means that many work on the basis of assumption and collusion. This means that partnership as a concept is not necessarily the most effective basis for effective teamwork. Case Study 27 exemplifies this.

Case Study 26

A registrar, Sue, in a four-partner practice was asked to carry out an audit of the appointments system because of the number of 'extras' the partners had to do as so-called emergency consultations. Sue found that they were 50 appointments short per week for the number of patient contacts to be expected. As a result, patients were waiting up to 14 days to see their own doctor if they did not say the matter was urgent. There was no practice standard for acceptable access in non-urgent cases. She recommended that more doctor time was needed. This was the outcome hoped for by three of the partners as they were feeling very stressed and overworked, so much so that they were prepared to take the necessary drop in income to accommodate a part-time additional partner.

The fourth partner, George, had always resisted more doctor time because he was unhappy at the idea of any drop in income. He felt that the price to be paid in terms of stress and workload was acceptable. Indeed, he was not really stressed now. He saw the audit as merely indicating that patient demand had gone up and that the same level of service could no longer be offered.

In carrying out the audit, Sue had noted that George had five-minute appointments, but always ran an hour or more late because each consultation took more than five minutes. He refused to lengthen his appointments. As a result he never did any extras. The registrar raised the issue with the partners, but they were not prepared to tackle George's clinical behaviour, even though it affected them. They preferred to keep the status quo rather than deal with the underlying behavioural issues, which were almost certainly the result of different philosophies and values. They decided to continue with the unsatisfactory service to patients and their own stress for the five years left before George retired.

As a result of the audit, they tinkered yet again with the working day, but no substantial change was achieved because they did not see, and therefore use, the link between the results of the audit and how they worked as a partnership.

Case Study 27

In a three-partner practice, the two senior partners, Richard and Ernest, shared responsibility for the finances and staff matters. Amazingly, the third partner, Luke, and the practice manager, Shirley, were kept in the dark about the details of the practice's finances, and the practice manager had to take all staff issues to Richard. Luke was very much the junior partner, and in any case was not interested in management issues as he saw them.

At the end of the practice's accounting year, insufficient money had been kept back to meet the tax bills, both of the practice and of the partners personally. At the same time, Richard had treated a poorly performing receptionist so badly that she was claiming constructive dismissal. Shirley had advised in writing that the steps Richard was taking were likely to be in breach of the employment contract, but he would not listen. When Shirley appealed to Luke for help in confronting Ernest over the financial muddle and Richard over the legal problems, Luke was unwilling to get involved. He could not see that he had shared responsibility with the others, and in particular enjoyed the present way of life too much to want to rock the boat. He saw that if he interfered or protested he would have to take more interest in the management of the practice, but more importantly he would have to stand up to not just one but both of the senior partners.

As a result, Shirley left to go to a bigger practice with more responsibility, the practice was dragged through an industrial tribunal and had to reinstate the receptionist with all the associated ignominy, and the next year the accountant told the partners to reduce their personal drawings by one-third to meet the tax debt. At this point, Luke started to confront Richard and Ernest, and with the help of the accountant and the practice solicitor began to make some headway. He found it too painful, however and eventually joined another practice where the need to confront seemed less acute.

HANDLING CONFLICT

Dysfunctional partnerships are major obstacles to corporate planning, decision making, teamworking and basic quality assurance. Dysfunctional partnerships often cannot decide because they do not know, and, if they do decide, they cannot implement because they dare not enforce. It follows that effective partnerships are open, honest and clear about their intentions and assumptions. However, openness and honesty carry with them a high risk of conflict. Conflict exists whenever an individual or group's interests diverge within an organization, or if its values or goals are at odds within itself. It is one of the key roles of management to understand the potential sources of conflict and to be able to predict how, when, and why they will arise.

Most partnerships know that conflict can arise from a clash of powerful personalities, uncertainty in the face of change and/or managerial versus clinical considerations. In the light of these likely sources of conflict, it is not surprising that there is a considerable amount of overt and covert tension within general practice. It is often the practice manager who perceives conflict and accurately predicts its likely impact on the organization. Reluctantly but wittingly the practice manager may have to sacrifice the interests of a single unit or part for the good of the whole. Case Study 28 gives an example of this.

Case Study 28

Brian Fuller was the new practice manager of a large, suburban practice that was becoming a fundholder somewhat reluctantly. It had had three new partners within a year (of whom one, Becky, was female), who joined four long-standing male partners. Brian had found the practice lacked personnel policies. There was no salary structure, no appraisal system, no regular communication process and no clarity of roles between the senior receptionist, the senior dispenser, the fundholding manager and the senior secretary.

Together with the partners Brian developed a clear plan of short-term changes and improvements to be made, particularly in relation to personnel matters. He agreed with the partners that there would be a hold on the longer term developments for the practice while he sorted the essentials for the staff. However, before he could proceed, the partnership found itself in crisis. The new partners, led by Becky, objected to the parity arrangements. Becky and David, the senior partner, had a violent row. It ended up with Becky and David shouting at each other, and David suggesting that Becky needed to see a psychiatrist about her inability to control her temper.

Brian, who had been present during the argument, spent the next six months, and most of his energy, trying to reconcile the two partners. He acted as go-between, shoulder to cry on, father confessor, teacher and calm influence. This helped all to decide whether they wanted to resolve the differences, however slowly and painfully, or whether they actually wanted to break up the partnership. However,

Case Study 28: *continued*

he was not able to get on with any of the planned staff changes, as the partners were unable to concentrate on anything except their potential split. The staff were very disappointed and felt very let down by Brian, who could not of course explain to them the problems. However, he was clear that his priority was to help resolve the conflict at the partnership level, which he eventually did. He was then able to get on with the staff matters.

Typical areas of conflict within general practice include differences of basic philosophies within the partnership (for instance whether or not to become fundholders), handling poor performance by a partner (for instance a partner who persistently fails to visit), handling a difficult member of staff, particularly and typically a long-serving practice manager and/or practice nurse (for instance when the staff member is a patient) or handling the place of external interests and activities within a practice (for example where one partner takes on outside commitments that will affect the practice without seeking approval first). These examples tell their own story, and probably ring many bells.

Much confusion arises because people concentrate on the 'how', or the implications of handling the conflict, instead of on the 'what' or the nature of the conflict itself. Case Study 29 exemplifies this.

Case Study 29

In a large urban practice, the practice manager had been in post for 23 years, working with the original partner as general factotum. As the practice grew so she grew with it, and took the title 'practice manager' very early. She was a patient of the practice. She was competent and knew the patients very well. She was not very skilled in handling staff, and was averse to change of any kind, which she saw as merely meaning more work.

As new partners joined the practice, her base became less secure and she became more obstructive and negative. The senior partner, who was her registered doctor, tried to defend her on all occasions, and several of the other long-serving staff, including the senior nurse, were supportive of her. They felt that she had given faithful service, and in any case her knowledge of the practice area and the individuals was vital to the health of the practice.

Cast Study 29: *continued*

The partners frequently complained about her among themselves. They felt frustrated and resentful. Yet whenever they arrived at exasperation point, they were held back because they dwelt immediately on the problems of getting rid of her. The patients would be up in arms, the other older staff would leave, she would make a fuss, and they would lose much vital information that only she knew. In addition, they kept wondering how they would replace her, and what this would mean for the work they would have to do in the management of the practice.

Eventually the partners called in a consultant, who pointed out to them that they needed to look at what sort of practice they wanted, and therefore articulate what sort of management such a practice would need. Only then could they decide how much of that management they wished to do themselves and how much they wished to delegate. From that would come a clear idea of the sort of skills and attributes they needed in a practice manager, against which they could measure their existing incumbent.

The message of this case study is that it is vital to stand back from issues (particularly if they are emotionally 'hot') and start by discussing the following questions:

- what sort of management decisions do the partners want to delegate?
- what sort of skills will this need?
- what sort of skills have they got?
- how big is the gap between where they are now and what they actually need?
- what sort of practice manager does the practice need?

When answers to these kind of questions become clear, then it is much easier to look at the options available to deal with a situation, and approach them objectively.

This is a useful approach for dealing with any conflict problems, especially those related to the partnership and its philosophy. Often the most difficult issues are about equity of workload and conflict arises when some partners feel overstressed by increased patient demand or are put upon when partners have outside appointments. Sometimes these problems can be resolved by extra appointments or running some extra surgeries, as we saw in Case Study 23. The underlying issues, however, are usually the nature of the increased patient demand. What is the evidence of changed behaviour on the part of either the doctors, the nurses or the patients themselves? Frequently the bottom line is insufficient overall clinical time for the patient demand. As we saw in Case Study 26, the options, therefore, are either to increase the clinical time by working harder or taking on a new partner, to delegate substantially by employing an assistant or nurse practitioner, to reduce the patient demand by closing the list, to reduce surgery times or to accept the pressure. All of these will have implications – the first ones will be financial – and unless those are worked through openly and honestly, then the conflicts will remain.

Issues and conflicts do not go away if they are ignored and not confronted. By the time they have become crises they are very 'hot' situations. There is no cool process in place. The art of managing conflict lies in anticipation, having protocols designed to deal with the 'what if'. Case Study 30 demonstrates this.

Guidelines and protocols were discussed earlier as part of clinical audit (Chapter 5). However, they are equally important as part of good management

Case Study 30

Penny was the youngest and newest partner in a five-partner practice. She had had maternity leave within two months of taking up her partnership, and when her child was two she decided to study for her MSc. She applied and was accepted, and then told the partners, with a request for the partnership to support her. She was looking for financial support, and agreement to time out for study and exams.

The partnership had nothing in its agreement to cover this, and no precedent. One partner, Miles, who had done a MD in his own time and at his own cost some 15 years ago, was adamant that this was not acceptable. Phil, the senior partner, was very irritated that Penny had not asked the partners first. However, the other partners were keen to support Penny, as one was pregnant, and another wanted to take on a clinical assistantship in the near future.

The practice had no agreed policy on time out for personal development by an individual partner, had no policy or budget for training and development across the partnership and an inadequate partnership agreement in relation to time out for pregnancy and/or partner training. Therefore, they had to decide on Penny's request while there was irritation and anger, anxiety and envy on the table.

It was Phil who eventually made the others see that they should decide on the policies they wanted to follow in relation to external activities, the level of support for individual development that the practice would sustain and in what circumstances, and revisit their partnership agreement, particularly what issues needed the partners'

Case Study 30: *continued*

prior agreement before further development. By taking this approach, the partners were able to find several matters within each category that needed policy decisions, thus taking the heat off the immediate problem of Penny's request.

As a result Penny was able to present her request within objective policies coolly agreed.

practice. They ensure that everybody is clear what will happen in given circumstances. They also ensure that there is a policy to follow that neutralizes and depersonalizes potentially difficult situations. Case Study 31 is such an example.

Case Study 31

A six-partner practice had an 'away day' at which, among other things, the issue of seniority and chairing the partnership was raised. There was no agreed senior partner – it was a concept that the practice had obdured for some time. Nevertheless, the oldest partner, Bill, always chaired the partnership and practice meetings, and tended to take decisions without consulting the others.

As a result of a full and frank discussion it was decided that the chair of the partnership should be appointed by annual election. No more than three consecutive years in office would be allowed. This protocol was agreed by all. Then the partnership elected Bill as chair.

After a year, no election had been held. One of the younger partners raised the issue privately with the practice manager, who brought the protocol to the attention of the practice meeting. Because an annual election was the agreed process, it was not seen as a threat to Bill, and no difficulty was caused. As he had performed well in the year, the practice re-elected him.

To handle conflict requires good leadership, good people and management skills and anticipation, all the major areas of high-level management that we have discussed so far. The same skills are needed to manage staff, as the next chapter shows.

12

Partners and staff – is this a team?

A society founded on individualism could fall apart without the glue of fraternity ... fraternity, or the awareness that there are others who are as important as oneself

Charles Handy

As we have seen general practitioners commonly find it difficult both to confront and to talk out issues within their partnership. It is not surprising therefore that they have the same problems with staff. Yet, as we have also seen, the partnership team must work for the rest of the practice to work. Indeed, the current trend of 'away days' for the whole practice is a fairly fruitless exercise if the partnership has not already had the opportunity to gain an understanding of the individual partners' agendas and to clarify the direction in which they all want to travel. As we have emphasized, the partners as employers have to set the organization's ambitions and direction and then sell them to the employees.

In so doing, however, they will undoubtedly take on board the views and ideas of their employees. According to Ghoshall and Bartlett:[2]

> Employees who share an organisation's ambitions and values have a far stronger incentive to collaborate than do employees whose sole incentives are financial.

Many relationship problems between boss and subordinates occur because bosses fail to make clear how they plan to use their authority and power. Recent evidence suggests that a disturbingly high proportion of practice teams do not function well.[3] The same writers also go on to say that this is particularly true when teams have no agreed objectives and that poor team-work is invariably part of a wider problem in which the management of a practice is in general terms deficient.

MOTIVATION

In looking to create a team with the staff, the partners must understand what motivates individuals to do their work. Hertzberg[4] has written extensively on the difference between *hygiene* factors and *motivating* factors. Hygiene factors are those sets of needs that can be seen as stemming from a human being's animal nature – the built-in drive to avoid pain from the environment, including drives such as hunger. The motivating factors are those that relate to the need to achieve and through achievement to experience psychological growth. Stimuli for the latter needs are the job content. Box 12.1 summarizes these two sets of factors.

Box 12.1   HYGIENE AND MOTIVATING FACTORS

Hygiene factors

- company policy
- administration
- supervision
- interpersonal relationships
- working conditions
- salary, status and security

Motivating factors

- achievement
- recognition for achievement
- the work itself
- responsibility
- growth or advancement

Motivating factors are the primary cause of satisfaction. Therefore it is very important to recognize that the provision of hygiene factors, upon which many employers concentrate, is insufficient to produce job satisfaction. Good conditions of service, good pay and efficient processes alone will not result in a contented and motivated workforce if there is no job satisfaction and responsibility. Case Study 32 demonstrates this.

The psychology of motivation is very complex, and what has been unravelled with any degree of assurance is very small indeed. But what is clear is that, in Hertzberg's words:

The surest and least circumlocutory way of getting someone to do something, is to kick him in the pants – give him what might be called KITA (a kick in the arse).

Case Study 32

A large, fundholding group practice had a small team of practice nurses, led by Barbara, who had ambitions to train as a nurse practitioner. The two part-time 'F'-grade nurses, Sheila and Sue, were anxious to develop their skills as well, in the areas of prevention. When the practice had decided to go into fundholding, the nurses had been very enthusiastic and supportive, as they saw it as their chance to develop themselves as well as the practice.

The practice was housed in a splendid purpose-built surgery, with excellent large treatment room facilities. The practice carried out minor surgery, but with the wife of one of the partners assisting. The practice did very little preventative work because the clinics were no longer reimbursed, and the partners felt that their income had fallen as a result of fundholding, while their workload had increased. They were not prepared to put money into developing the nurses' services as they saw that as a route to increased pay demands.

When the nurses complained about the heavy workload and no development, the partners decided to take on a nursing auxiliary straight from school. She was very cheap and quickly learned the basics of phlebotomy and how to apply simple dressings. The nurses were furious as they had not been consulted, and were anxious that the doctors might see this as a way of reducing trained nurse time.

The relationships got worse, as the nurses felt undervalued and underused. Eventually Barbara was successful in getting another post locally at a practice that specifically wanted to train a nurse practitioner. The partners did not replace her at 'G' grade but brought in another nursing auxiliary and another part-time nurse. The result was a highly demotivated group of staff, working in good conditions, and ill-feeling that spread to other parts of the surgery.

Hertzberg also goes on to say that, in what he calls negative psychological KITA,

the cruelty is not visible. The bleeding is internal and comes much later. It reduces the possibility of physical backlash. Since the number of psychological pains that a person can feel is almost infinite, the direction and site possibilities of the KITA are increased many times. The person administering the kick can manage to be above it all and let the system accomplish the dirty work. Those who practice it receive some ego satisfaction (one-upmanship) whereas they would find drawing blood abhorrent.

Lastly, if an employee does complain he or she can always be accused of being paranoid, since there is no tangible evidence of attack.

This mode of management does not lead to motivation but merely to movement in one direction or another. The best, and all too common, example of this is harassment or bullying of receptionists by partners in the full glare of the waiting room, as was shown in Case Study 20.

One of the biggest problems for doctors in fulfilling their management motivational role in general practice lies in the complex part that they play in the workforce team. As we noted in Chapter 10, they are not only the employers with a separate organizational framework called the partnership, but they are also the face workers upon whose efforts the success of the practice largely relies. Their support teams, the reception, nursing and administrative teams, would ideally need to have supervisory control, or certainly effective management, of the work of the doctors in the consulting room to be maximally motivated and to ensure maximally efficient use of resources. Because of the dual role of the doctors as partners and as face workers, this is clearly not possible, and tensions arise. Doctors, because of the narrowness generally of their medical education, have little experience of the pressures and stresses attaching to other members of the practice team. Recently, they have become preoccupied with their own stress, which seems to have accentuated this. The partners are also focused on the consulting room and therefore upon themselves and their skills. There is regrettably still wide experience of doctors not according other members of the practice team (particularly of the female gender) the respect and understanding that they would give to medical colleagues. This is a major demotivating factor for non-clinical members of the primary health care team.

For all these reasons, therefore, doctors as managers tend not to exercise their management responsibilities to satisfy such motivations. This is a serious problem because, as Ghoshall and Bartlett[2] put it:

> At the foundation of an institution entrepreneurial process is a culture that sets great store by the ability of the individual.

The two other areas that cause most difficulties in terms of the handling of people are:

- delegation
- error.

DELEGATION

Delegation is a means of extending one's own competence by the competencies of others, and the best delegation is to people who have skills beyond oneself. Delegation is not a way of passing the buck, or 'dumping'! It is vital to delegate well whether to a clinical colleague or as part of the practice management function.

Managers, particularly those in complex organizations such as general practices, cannot perform by themselves all the tasks necessary for success. They must manage others in order to perform, and they must be willing to do so without seeking immediate and personal feedback.

The art of good delegation is to be clear about what is expected of the delegatee, what role that person is being asked to assume in solving a particular problem. They must be given the appropriate authority and resources to carry out that task and offered the appropriate amount of support to carry it out. Box 12.2 sets out the rules of good delegation.

Box 12.2   RULES FOR GOOD DELEGATION[5]

- Never do work that others can do. Ask whether it could be done by somebody else, whether it could be done more quickly some other way, whether it could be done more effectively at some other time or whether it needs to be done at all.
- Always think carefully about the purpose of the delegation. If it is not clear, then the person to whom the work is being delegated has little hope of understanding the reason for the act of delegation. To be successful the purpose needs to be established, then the relevant people need to be told what tasks are involved, what is expected of them, and what constitutes effective performance.
- Make sure that the person to whom the task or responsibility is being delegated knows and agrees with the arrangements and timescale for control and monitoring.
- If it has been said that the whole job is being delegated, then it is important that no part is being kept quietly back. If it is, and comes to light later, it would indicate a lack of trust: it often means that the most interesting part of the task is being retained.
- Make sure that there are adequate resources available to carry out the tasks and plan to provide these in advance. They may include training or giving experience, or examining how the work fits with the other work that the individual is doing.
- Make sure that the delegatee understands what is required by using language that is clear and free from technical jargon. Bear in mind that any messages passed on by word of mouth are subject to involuntary distortion.
- If a mistake arises in a delegated task, criticism should always be constructive and in private. Make sure that the process of delegation was correct, before pursuing further assessment of fault or blame.

Box 12.2: *continued*

- Ask whether there is anything more that could be delegated, particularly to the practice nurse, district nurse and health visitor.
- Responsibility for a task cannot be delegated, particularly where legal accountability is involved. The delegatee can be made accountable to the delegator for the delegated task, but the delegator cannot duck out of final responsibility.

A manager's democracy is not measured by the number of decisions subordinates make. The sheer number of the decisions is not an accurate index. More important is the significance of the decisions.[6]

Handling error

> Mistakes will be made but if a person is essentially right, the mistakes that he or she makes are not nearly as serious in the long run as the mistakes management will make if it is dictatorial and undertakes to tell those under its authority how they must do their jobs.
>
> *William McKnights, 3M's Chairman and Chief Executive*

The above quotation sums it up. The good handling of error is a sign of a mature and well-managed organization. All mistakes are opportunities to learn.

Creating the sort of environment where this is true is vital to ensure employees feel not only that the organization is fair, but that they can have confidence that those with whom they share responsibility will contribute equitably. A well-established sense of fairness serves as an organizational safety net for those of the staff who feel they want to take some risk and use some initiative. Case Study 33 illustrates this.

Much of that sense of fairness can be enshrined in written codes of conduct and disciplinary and grievance procedures. These are particularly powerful when they are developed and agreed by staff and arise out of a generally accepted need to take further the concept of no one being surprised by events (Chapter 9). It is always a mistake to develop such procedures in a 'hot 'and isolated situation. It creates a much greater confidence in the innate fairness of the organization if such procedures can be part of an overall exercise looking at potential scenarios and protocols to handle them.

A frequent cry from doctors is 'nothing happens unless we initiate it'. Often this is because staff are concerned that if they initiate something, that is if they take a risk, they will not be fairly treated and, if the initiative turns out to

Case Study 33

In a five-partner inner city practice, the partners held weekly staff meetings to give and exchange information about the developments in all parts of the practice. One week they discussed the advantages and disadvantages of opportunistic management of chronic conditions, and the receptionists and nurses were enthusiastic about trying a more organized way of working through the 'at-risk' groups. The partners were happy for them to work up proposals.

The three members of the practice nurse team each took a chronic condition – asthma, diabetes, hypertension – and read up on it, including information about courses and training, costs and timescales. They planned the order in which they could do the relevant training, and agreed they would each cover the consequent absences. They took their ideas to the receptionists and the practice manager, to add in their administrative proposals for running the clinics. They then took their options to the partners, who were happy to endorse the proposals.

Stimulated by this, the practice secretary was enthused to develop her ideas about setting up preformatted forms for referral requests and a system for maintaining data in this area for audit purposes. The partners found themselves with staff who were brimming over with ideas for developing patient services.

be a mistake, that they will be 'punished'. Case Study 34 provides such an example.

The failure to use mistakes as a learning opportunity for both the individual and the organization tends to erode any kind of use of initiative or entrepreneurial activity at all levels. The practice manager, the leader of the staff team, will certainly feel demotivated and demoralized if all errors and mistakes are laid at his or her door. Such 'mistakes' could range from failure to pick up the rubbish from the car park to producing surprising and unwelcome end of year financial figures for the partnership. The practice manager will in turn pass on that attitude to colleagues and subordinates.

Delegation, as we saw earlier, requires an ability to handle error. Asking other people to do things that you cannot because of lack of time or skill is a high-risk enterprise. The result may be performance that is less than if you had done the task yourself. General practice culture, because of the element of 'life and death' is not one that is comfortable with that concept. The reverse, however, is to trust people to be appropriately motivated and train them to do the work.

Case Study 34

John and Ernest were the two partners in a small rural practice. Both were single-handed general practitioners at heart, and resented each other and the fact that they had to delegate some activities to staff. They both, but particularly Ernest, denigrated the efforts of the practice nurse and senior receptionist to make improvements to the rather limited environment for care that their practice offered. Jean, the practice nurse, suggested a system for improving waiting times for diabetic patients with routine repeat appointments. Ernest refused to discuss what he described as a 'stupid idea' that would only add to his workload. It required him to suggest to the patient that when they returned for a check-up they saw the practice nurse first to have their blood pressure and urine sample taken.

As a result, the practice nurse never made any suggestions again, and this lack of initiative rubbed off on the other staff. When John actually asked for ideas about the appointments system, no one offered any. This merely fuelled his belief that, if any ideas were needed, the doctors would have to come up with them.

THE PRACTICE MANAGER

It is worthwhile taking time here to look at the role of the practice manager in the creation and development of the staff team. The first problem lies in the ambiguity of the role and the discomfort of the position, sitting as it were in the neck of the hourglass between the owners of the practice, who are also the coalface workers, and the rest of the practice team.

The practice manager is a hybrid creature, ranging from little more than a senior receptionist, doing all the jobs that the partners find too tedious, through to a group business manager, particularly in fundholding practices, with a 'seat on the board' and, in rare cases, a partnership share. The ambiguity lies in the manager as a member of the partner team, which is essentially a contractual and legal convenience, and being the chief executive of the organization, working to a board of directors (the doctors), and being responsible for the overall performance of the practice to that board.

A few practice managers have taken the leap and become some kind of partner. Very few hold shares or share profit and salary. The issue of common liability for medical negligence is rarely thought through. The important relationship is that between the practice manager – as an employee and as chief executive to the board – and the support staff. Janus-headed, the manager sits as the repository of all information, the receiver of all complaints and brick bats, the miracle worker and ringmaster. When used effectively, practice managers are an enormous source of skill and competence to whom the partnership can delegate those parts of the management of the practice at which they are not skilled. The many case studies in this book illustrate all these roles.

There has been rapid growth in numbers and increase in the quality of practice managers in the last ten years. Fundholding has had a major impact upon both the salary offered and the skills demanded. Much of the detailed day-to-day management and management competencies can be safely left to a well-qualified practice manager. Such a practice manager will be a key contributor to strategic issues as well – looking ahead and achieving a sense of direction. They frequently handle conflict, and it is the practice manager who can often act as the arbiter and go-between in partnership disputes. It can be a lonely and complex job, and partners should not forget the sustaining, training and development needs of their principal member of staff (see Chapter 13).

CONCLUSION

It is important when ensuring appropriate delegation and understanding people's motivation that this is not dumping, or pandering to individuals' needs to a point where the organizational needs are forgotten. Creating an effective team means balancing the personal growth of subordinates with organizational efficiency, and, at the end of the day, patients' needs.

Important as teamwork is, like communication, it is not something that, of itself (even if improved), will achieve good management. It is only in relation to the overall health of the practice that improvements in these particular areas will make any difference. Development and training is of major importance because of the role it plays in helping people understand what Glouberman and Mintzberg[7] call 'the other actors in the system'. Ensuring effective delegation and reducing the amount of error is of itself a major reason for investing appropriately in development and training. All too frequently this sort of investment goes by the board. Moreover, it is also a sign of respect for the individual and an intrinsic part of the motivational factors that make people feel self-disciplined and committed. Furthermore, it is important in a book on quality assurance to pay suitable attention to the overall place of training and development for the whole of the practice team. We develop this in the next chapter.

REFERENCES

1   Handy C (1989) *The Age of Unreason*. London: Hutchinson.

2   Ghoshall S, Bartlett C A (1995) Changing the role of top management. *Harvard Business Review*; Jan/Feb: 86–96.

3   West M, Poulton B, Hardy G (1995) *New Models of Primary Health Care: the Northern and Yorkshire Region Micro-purchasing Project*. Leeds: NYRHA.

4   Hertzberg F (1966) *Work and the Nature of Man*. New York: World Publishing.

5   Irvine S (1992) *Balancing Dreams and Discipline*. London: RCGP.

6   Drucker P (1995) The information executives truly need. *Harvard Business Review*; Jan/Feb: 54–62.

7   Glouberman S, Mintzberg H (1994) *Managing the Care of Health and the Cure of Disease*. Paper presented to King's Fund Seminar.

13

Learning for quality

Medical education is a reflection of medical practice; it is not the education that will change the practitioners, but reformed practice that will redesign medical education

Silver (1983)[1]

Skilled people are a practice's gold in the bank, the foundation that, if sound, will enable it to flourish. A practice's managers therefore have a primary responsibility to use a practice's human resources effectively. So partnerships must begin to view training, education and professional development, and the accountability of individuals to the practice for their competence and performance, as essential elements of practice business. The starting point is a professional and practice culture that actively promotes learning and excellence of performance.[2,3] Few practices operate this way today, so this is new ground.

This chapter looks at ways of creating a learning culture, underpinned by a practice strategy and programme for education and continuing professional development.

ESTABLISHING THE CULTURE

Establishing a learning culture in any organization starts at the top. So it will fall to the partners, as the owners, to create the culture and to show that they practice what they preach and that they are willing to find the means of nurturing and supporting it for themselves and others. In education, as in other aspects of practice, leadership by partners is fundamental (Chapter 11). It would be extremely difficult for other members of the practice team to introduce the learning culture without a positive and unreserved commitment from the partners.

And what is this culture? It has to be founded on a practice's ethos, values and standards. A culture based on learning will be open, outward-looking, inquisitive, questioning, always 'seeking after the truth'. It will welcome new knowledge, respect evidence, be analytical and understand the relationship between research, practice and education. The learning practice will want and be able to learn from experience, both its own and others. It will see self-criticism and testing against others as strengths. Consequently, it will give permission to its members to make mistakes provided they learn how to get it right next time. The learning practice will celebrate good practice and seek excellence through sustained, incremental improvement.

Obstacles to overcome

There will be difficulties to overcome. First, general practitioners have had a remarkably individualistic approach to their own training and education, based on the premise that each person can be relied upon to decide whether, what and how much should be learnt for safe practice. Second, there is ambivalence towards objective assessment, to testing against others. Third, there appears to be a reluctance generally to use the principles of adult learning and techniques that facilitate learning such as significant event analysis and clinical audit (Chapter 4). Finally, there is a passive attitude to confronting poor practice.

Because partnerships are often ambivalent about their responsibilities for their own education and performance, they can be equally ambivalent in providing for the training and continuing education for people who they employ. Consequently it has been health authorities rather than general practitioners who have tended to take the lead in establishing systematic training at the practice level for receptionists, secretaries, practice nurses and others. It is still quite exceptional, for example, for a practice partnership to set out the nursing requirements of a practice clearly, and from that to derive the skills and competencies required for individuals and the nursing team as a whole. Case Study 35 illustrates the problem.

Case Study 35

The Frost Medical Practice was taking on a new practice nurse. The partners felt that they needed one, although they were not quite sure what the person would do. They had no specific plan or future policies for the nursing area, or an analysis of skills needed. They had decided that the definition of the job would have to wait until the partners saw what the nurse joining them could actually do! When one arrived, the partners discovered that her real interest lay in becoming a nurse practitioner, and the practice had no plans or resources to develop this. She left.

A PRACTICE TRAINING PROGRAMME

The period of *laissez-faire* is now ending. To identify its educational needs thoroughly a practice must have a clear idea of its aims and future plans (Chapter 8). Any practice plan that realistically attempts to look forward, to establish a set of objectives for the forthcoming year or years, has to include a review of the knowledge and skills required to achieve those objectives. The practice must then review the skills and experience that the existing team possesses, and then work out how to fill the gaps. Training, education and professional development are becoming more formal and structured, and more clearly related to the work that people are actually expected to do, be they doctors, nurses, managers or administrative staff.

In a modern practice the costs of training and development are considerable in terms of course and training fees and loss of remunerated time to the practice, and also in terms of disturbance and stress on those covering for the person being trained. So, to manage a practice educational programme successfully it is important to plan ahead. The training and continuing professional development of all staff need to be coordinated and focused. It helps if one senior member of the practice, reporting to the partnership, is given responsibility for overseeing the practice's educational strategy and programme. Then a named person can be held accountable for ensuring that partnership and practice team decisions on educational matters are well informed and properly implemented.

The practice training programme should be one of the most effective weapons in the armoury for developing quality care. It should answer the following questions (Box 13.1).

Box 13.1   PRACTICE TRAINING PROGRAMME

- who needs to be trained?
- what do they need to be trained in or for? (i.e. the training subject)
- how do they need to be trained? (i.e. the training method)
- when will they be trained?
- how much will it cost?
- what are the priorities?

Adapted from Irvine and Haman[4]

A coherent, viable programme will be based on the principles of adult learning. It will include:

- a clear statement of the practice's educational aims and objectives, derived from the practice development plan

- an agreed plan of educational activities and priorities
- clarity about the range of knowledge and skills each practice function requires
- clarity in understanding of the roles of all individual practice members.

Thus, the range of knowledge and skills required for posts in the practice should be explicit and published to all the team's members. Clarity is one of the key ways of ensuring a healthy team (Chapter 10) and preventing conflict and tension (Chapter 11).

An early task for the person in charge of the programme is to talk with each post-holder – partners, nurses and others – to assess their perception of their skills and learning needs against the requirements of the job and the future plans of the practice. Box 13.2 lists the sorts of questions such an interview should cover.

Box 13.2   QUESTIONS FOR TRAINING INTERVIEW

- what do I need to know to do my job?
- what do I need to know to do my job in the future?
- what do I need to know for my own satisfaction?
- which parts of my job take up most of the time?
- which parts of my job do I find most worrying or difficult?
- what in my job would I like to do better?
- are there any factors which hinder me in carrying out my job?
- do I have skills which I could impart to other members of the practice that would help them in their jobs?

Some practices do this. They use the practice development plan (Chapter 9) as the strategic policy instrument, and work back from that to determine what their overall skill mix and general educational needs are to achieve their purpose. Then they customize the plan to individual posts in the practice. They use appraisal interviews, clinical guidelines and the results of clinical and organizational audit to identify gaps in competence and performance in the organization and in individuals within. In this way their resulting educational programmes are dynamic, relevant and always adjusting to the practice's and individual's changing needs.

Practices working in this way know where the money comes from to fund established educational commitments, and may well be prepared to assign funds of their own to complement these, as Case Study 36 illustrates.

Case Study 36   Staff Training and Development[5]

A fundholding general practice assigned £10 000 worth of savings to establish a practice educational fund. This fund, administered by the partner responsible for training, was to be used to help members of the practice pay for educational activities that were deemed to be furthering the objectives of the practice, and which could not be supported from other sources. Examples of practice educational activities supported this way included:

- one partner attending a diploma course in therapeutics in order to take overall responsibility for practice prescribing
- two partners strengthening their management skills, one by joining an MBA course and the other an Open University course in health services management
- a trainee nurse practitioner undertaking an honours degree course for nurse practitioners
- the practice manager undertaking a diploma course in business administration
- a receptionist attending a new skills course
- an enrolled nurse on a conversion course to become an RGN
- a health visitor taking study days to develop skills in health needs assessment

Practices with an educational programme will have more opportunities for introducing shared learning. For example, a practice introducing a new clinical guideline will want to be sure that all clinicians involved in such care – nurses as well as doctors – are knowledgeable about the subject. So there is, immediately, a substantial educational opportunity when converting a national guideline for practice purposes to a form suitable for the practice, using a practice 'guidelines group' as suggested in Chapter 5. The wider practice team can learn about the clinical content of newly created practice guidelines by attending lectures together or by practice-based seminars. Shared learning in these circumstances, as a means of knowledge transfer and as a teambuilder, tends to work well because the participants have a common purpose: the care of their patients. It encourages personal reading and writing, which are still central to effective learning.

PERSONAL DEVELOPMENT/APPRAISAL

Good training and good continuing education go hand in hand with personal development. Development has two sides to it: the development of the job and the development of the individual. The former can be achieved by enriching the job, which may provide the opportunity for the employee's psychological growth, by making the activity more interesting and responsible. Job development needs care to maintain a balance between development of the individual as a person and merely adding to that person's workload.

The development of the individual can be best addressed by the use of an effective appraisal system, which of itself should be a central plank of any practice's quality control arrangements.[4] Regular performance appraisal, including appraisal of partner by partner, must surely become part of continuing professional development. It should be seen as a formative method which can help individuals find out how they might best develop themselves and overcome recognized problems. And appraisal interviews chart the way forward for each team member through their plans for their own personal development. It is the basis of portfolio learning and provides the baseline for subsequent review.[6]

Experience shows that most non-medical people think that performance appraisal is a good idea. The concerns often lie in the practicalities of implementation. According to Ovreteit:[7]

> In listening to a subordinate's review of performance, problems and failings the manager is automatically cast in the role of counsellor. This role for the manager in turn results naturally in a problem-solving discussion. In the traditional performance appraisal interview, on the other hand, the manager is automatically cast in the role of judge.

MEETING THE TRAINING NEEDS

The change in direction towards adult learning in practice, supported by effective appraisal and other aids, is beginning to show in the ways in which the main professions represented in the practice team are responding. We briefly summarize these below.

General practitioners

Several new developments should focus educational provision to enhance the quality of practice education:

- objective assessment as a requirement for the certification of vocational training

- voluntary higher training as part of further professional development.[3,8,9] For example the Postgraduate Institute at the University of Newcastle upon Tyne introduced a Diploma in Advanced General Practice in 1995, specifically designed to give further knowledge and skills in management, quality assurance, the epidemiology required for health status and health needs assessment and research appraisal. The purpose is to close the skills gap between what is expected of general practitioners to make a modern practice work and what vocational training equips doctors to do now
- a more structured approach to personal professional development, with the use of portfolio learning, mentoring, personal appraisal and personal development plans and continuing education directed to continuing effectiveness[10,11]
- an exploration of some regular assessment of the performance of the established practitioner.

Underpinning these developments are moves to strengthen the infrastructure of the education of general practitioners, partly by cementing closer working relationships between university departments of general practice and the university postgraduate organizations and partly by the development of local tutorial arrangements from which mentoring can flow.[12]

Nurses

The UK Central Council for Nursing, Health Visiting and Midwifery (UKCC) has recently introduced new arrangements for Post-registration Education and Practice (PREP) of all nurses. The PREP programme requires trained nurses to demonstrate learning and changed clinical practice through portfolio learning.

The key elements of continuing education and further professional development for nurses in the community were described recently by the NHS Management Executive.[13] Nurses should participate in continuing education that:

- meets contemporary health needs and the demands of service provision and conforms to the UKCC standards framework
- is suited to the area of clinical practice in which the primary health care nurse is working
- is based on, and set in, the clinical practice arena where new knowledge can be generated to bring about change in nursing.

Practice managers

In the past, practice managers have had very little formal educational provision. Investment in training and continuing education has been introduced only recently, when health authorities began to recognize the need for more effective support.

The professional body for practice managers, the Association of Managers in General Practice (AMGP), has developed significant training programmes in this area. It has explicit standards and lays down competencies expected of practitioners in practice management who wish to achieve certificate and diploma status, and relates these to nationally accepted standards, both National Vocational Training Qualifications (NVCQ) and Management Charter Initiative (MCI) standards of competence for managers.[14]

As we saw in Chapter 12, some practices, under the stimulus of fund-holding, have begun to close the knowledge and skills gap in their practices by recruiting managers with appropriate skills and external training. Management qualifications, such as diplomas in management studies, MBAs, as well as the specialist diplomas of AMGP and the Institute of Health Service Management, are common requirements.

Receptionists and secretaries

The arrangements for the initial training and further education of secretaries and receptionists in general practice have been patchy, in spite of the sterling work done by organizations such as the Association of Medical Secretaries, Practice Administrators and Receptionists and the Joint Committee for Education of Practice Administrators and Secretarial Staff. Their support for initiatives such as the Practice Receptionist Programme[15] provided an incentive to health authorities, who have begun to see it as one of their responsibilities to try and improve competence and performance in this sector. This has taken the form mainly of release to specific courses or training days, often run by FHSAs themselves. Building on this, a growing number of practices now look to in-house training, and make time available for this.

CONCLUSION

A practice that can cultivate an attitude, a climate and culture which values learning, and which actively and openly appreciates and supports the seeking of high standards of practice by individual members, will have perhaps the most important building block of quality practice firmly in place. Regular education informed by the results of regular performance monitoring through clinical audit and personal appraisal are the keys to maintaining competence and performance in individual practitioners. Practices cannot afford to neglect or ignore this function.

REFERENCES

1   Silver G A (1983) Victim or villain. *Lancet*; **ii**: 960.

2   Schön D A (1979) Public service organisations and the capacity for public learning. *International Social Science Journal*; **xxxi**: 683–94.

3   Irvine D H (1993) General practice in the 1990s: a personal view of future developments. *British Journal of General Practice*; **43**: 121–5.

4   Irvine S, Haman H (1993) *Making Sense of Personnel Management*. Oxford: Radcliffe Medical Press.

5   Lintonville Medical Group (1993) Ashington, Northumberland. Personal communication.

6   Royal College of General Practitioners (1993) *Portfolio-based Learning in General Practice*. Occasional Paper No 63. London: RCGP.

7   Ovreteit J (1992) *Health Service Quality*. Oxford: Blackwell Special Projects.

8   Royal College of General Practitioners (1990) Educational strategy for general practice for the 1990s. In *A College Plan. Priorities for the Future*. Occasional Paper 49. London: RCGP.

9   Koppell I, Pietroni R G (1991) *Higher Professional Education Causes in the United Kingdom*. Occasional Paper 51. London: RCGP.

10 Royal College of General Practitioners (1994) *Education and Training for General Practice*. Policy Statement 3. London: RCGP.

11 National Association of Health Authorities and Trusts (1994) *Partners in Learning: Developing Postgraduate Training and Continuing Education for General Practice*. London: NAHAT.

12 Standing Committee on Postgraduate Medical and Dental Education (1994) *Continuing Professional Development for Doctors and Dentists*. London: SCOPME.

13 NHS Management Executive (1993) *Nursing in Primary Health Care: New World, New Opportunities*. London: NHSE.

14 Association of Managers in General Practice (1994) *General Medical Practice Management*. Bristol: NHS Training Directorate.

15 Radcliffe Medical Press (1995) *Practice Receptionists Programme* 1 and 2. Oxford: Radcliffe Medical Press.

The Role of External Review in Quality

14

The regulatory framework

Prevention is better than cure

There are two basic approaches to assuring quality. The first is what people in a practice do themselves. The second is the external framework of professional regulation and contract. We believe that the more practices can succeed unaided, the less reason there is for elaborate outside controls which people dislike.

This chapter outlines the professional framework. Today, professional bodies are giving more attention to the performance of career health professionals. We touch, therefore, on the policy issues surrounding recertification and reaccreditation.

DEFINITIONS

The language is a terminological minefield. Terms such as 'certification' and 'accreditation' are bandied about, causing confusion. To try and avoid further confusion, we will first explain the meaning of terms used here so that at least our readers should be clear!

Licensure

Licensure is defined as 'formal permission from a constituted authority to do something' (*Shorter Oxford English Dictionary*, 1973). In the UK the national medical and nursing licensing bodies are the General Medical Council (GMC) and the UKCC. Each has a statutory basis for its authority. Each is entrusted by society to ensure that only properly qualified people are allowed to practice. Licensing bodies, in protecting the public, have the right to suspend or remove practitioners for professional misconduct or incompetence.

Registration

The national licensing bodies implement their statutory functions by maintaining registers of practitioners who they have licensed to practice. Being registered gives doctors and nurses the right to practice, to earn a livelihood from their profession. Registration carries with it duties and obligations that a practitioner is expected to meet. Both Councils give guidance about its nature.

Certification

The term 'certification' indicates the completion of a period of post-registration training. Certification can simply denote attendance at a training programme or 'the formal definition of a practitioner's competence and performance'.[1] It is this latter usage that is most common because people want to be sure that in the future a 'certificated' practitioner is safe.

Certification, once achieved, cannot subsequently be taken away. Time-limited certification is therefore used when the certificating body believes that its assessments have limited predictive value, mainly because the content and nature of practice changes fairly quickly. This is why, for example, the American Board of Family Practice (the equivalent of the Joint Committee on Postgraduate Training for General Practice (JCPTGP)) limits its certification to seven years. Time-limited certification is therefore a precondition of any form of recertification.[2]

Recertification

Recertification is the process by which a professional body 'testifies intermittently to the competence of each of its members, either with or without a period of formal retraining'.[2]

Accreditation

The term 'accreditation' is used in three ways in general practice today.

First, it is 'the formal recognition and attestation of a standard of quality achieved by a general practice',[1] hence 'practice accreditation'. Second, it is used as an alternative to 'certification'. Third, it can denote an approved training programme or educational experience. We use the first, the RCGP terminology.

Practice accreditation is invariably time limited. Indeed, it is usually so.

Approved

The term 'approved' normally describes a recognized educational experience – a hospital post approved for training or a course approved for the postgraduate education allowance (PGEA).

So, to summarize, we say that:

- *certificated* refers to the individual
- *accredited* refers to the practice
- *approved* refers to an educational experience.

Competence and performance

It is essential to distinguish between competence and performance, for often these terms are also used interchangeably. Lloyd[3] offers the following definition:

- *competence* – what a practitioner is capable of doing
- *performance* – what a practitioner does in practice.

Competence and performance should therefore be considered as separate constructs.[4] The competent practitioner has the knowledge, skills and attitudes necessary for effective practice. Performance is the application of knowledge and skills in practice. Established practitioners emphasize performance because it reflects their everyday work. Nevertheless, performance is substantially dependent on competence. A competent practitioner may have an off-day, and so perform inadequately; but an incompetent practitioner can never perform consistently well. Assessments of performance, to be valid, must therefore include assessments of competence.

CHANGING IDEAS ABOUT ACCOUNTABILITY

Professionals like to supervise their own standards. Professional bodies see it as their responsibility to define training and continuing education, and to make sure that newcomers to a profession are competent. Accountability for the competence of members is at the heart of self-regulating professions.

The public's previously unquestioning trust that doctors and nurses must be safe because they are 'qualified' is being replaced by expectations of more explicit assurance on continuing professional performance. This development is challenging for professionals and their regulating bodies. It is why professional bodies are now extending their remit from competence – essentially educational – to include performance.

Certification on completion of training is an accepted and respected part of the regulatory framework, and we need say no more about it. But practice accreditation and recertification, and the need for arrangements to deal with poorly performing doctors, are new, and are discussed further.

PRACTICE EXTERNAL REVIEW

It is easiest to start by looking at the current approaches to periodic practice external review. These are summarized in Table 14.1.

We describe the methods in full in Chapter 15 alongside the case histories that illustrate them. Some are awards, some for selective accreditation; some are mainly about an individual, some primarily about aspects of the practice.

Table 14.1   Approaches to practice external review

Method	Practice or individual	Purpose
JCPT/RCGP (Teaching Practice)	Trainer/teaching practice selection	Accreditation
RCGP Fellowship by Assessment	Individual/practice	Award
BS5750/BS EN ISO 9000	Practice	Accreditation
King's Fund Organisational Audit	Practice	Accreditation
Investors in People	Practice	Accreditation
Charter Mark	Practice	Award

Purpose of external review

Being clear about purpose, and therefore about motivation, is extremely important. Practice external review may have several functions:

- to demonstrate the achievement of defined standards to the outside world
- to stimulate practices to improve
- to give practices the status and sense of satisfaction that stems from achieving standards which they value

- to enable practices to explore new opportunities, take on further responsibilities (such as teaching) or provide additional services (such as minor surgery)
- to provide the public and health commissioners with evidence of quality.

Practice external review provides a major stimulus for practices that want voluntarily to try and match themselves against an external standard (Chapter 3). But it is more than this. Practices that have gone through review invariably say that, as for any inspection, the main value lies in the preparation itself rather than in the accolade at the end. Preparation for practice external review can thus be a major opportunity for learning, an important aid to teambuilding and a promoter of confidence and therefore high morale.[5] This view is certainly shared by the practitioners whose experiences are described in Chapter 15.

Professional bodies may use external review as the basis of practice accreditation. The best example of this use is the long-standing 'accrediting' of practices for teaching purposes by the RCGP and JCPTGP working through the university post-graduate organizations.

With rising consumer awareness, patients are increasingly likely to ask whether the practice they propose to join has been reviewed and accredited by a reputable agency. Accreditation is becoming equated in the public mind with standards, and the public as users of health care are becoming more conscious of standards in an era of patient charters, league tables and consumer guides.

Health commissions are also interested in practice accreditation. They act for patients. If practice accreditation is based on parameters which are right for them, then they are likely to use it. This is the reason why many health commissions and community trusts are sponsoring practices for external review.[6]

General characteristics of accreditation

A valid practice accreditation will:

- seek to promote improvement
- be professionally led
- be based on explicit standards
- be comprehensive
- demonstrate compliance with standards
- include verification by inspection
- be conducted by an independent agency.

Promote improvement

Accreditation based on inspection is frequently criticized because it is said to encourage minimalist behaviour: 'all we need to do is to show that we did the right things on the day'. This is is a very restrictive approach and probably ineffective. Accreditation can and should be positive, to stimulate improvement for patients and practitioners. That is exactly what today's methods try to do.

Ovretveit[7] says that, for accreditation to have a predictive value, it must ask practices to show that they have effective quality systems. Sustained improvement is not achievable in a practice without the desire and capacity to learn, and the systems to translate commitment into action.

Peer led

The professions have to have a significant say in determining and monitoring standards – ownership and commitment go hand in hand. Peers should be the best judges of what is technically desirable and in knowing whether compliance is thorough.

Users must also be involved. For example, vocational registrars – as recipients of training – may take part in teaching practice reaccreditation by giving feedback and being represented on trainer reappointment committees. There has been patient involvement in creating the standards for the King's Fund Organisational Audit (KFOA). And the assessors for General Practice Quality Assured (GPQA), KFOA and Investors in People include 'lay' people.

Be comprehensive

All existing methods are incomplete. But ideally accreditation should be comprehensive. Comprehensiveness does not mean that everything has to be assessed. Judicious sampling is likely to be the most feasible way of building up a representative picture of a practice.

Based on explicit standards

This has been relatively easy to accomplish with the methods in use today because they concentrate on the organizational and environmental characteristics for which criteria of quality can be specified easily and measured accurately. Standards of access to the doctor, waiting times for patients and effective appointment systems are examples.

Looking ahead, clinical aspects will be involved. Observing the use of clinical guidelines, effective prescribing and sound risk management procedures are examples of practice whose clinical quality can be assessed. There are also those subjective but nevertheless important aspects of patient care, for example helpfulness, good communication and responsiveness, which will not yield easily to measurement yet must be accounted for in the reckoning.

Inspection

All methods in use today rely on some form of inspection supported by documentation. Some use external standards while others want practices to comply with their own, internally generated standards.

Independent

There is some speculation today about who the accrediting agency should be. There can be more than one. The JCPTGP/RCGP/postgraduate organization complex is the longest established. Since the purpose is teaching, the choice of a professional agency is appropriate. The King's Fund Organisational Audit and the British Standards Institution are independent of provider affiliation. Independence has advantages (Box 14.1).

Box 14.1   ADVANTAGES OF INDEPENDENT ACCREDITING AGENCIES

- they are independent of providers and purchasers and pressure groups
- they should put the interests of patients (or registrars) first
- in terms of standards, they are best placed to reconcile the perspectives of the various stakeholders, including the professions, patients, commissioners and tax-payers
- as national agencies, they can apply national standards and so seek to reduce inappropriate national and local variation
- they should develop a consistency of method, so to produce comparative data whose quality and integrity can be assured

---

Summary

Practice external review provides an excellent foundation for the development of fully comprehensive practice accreditation. The gaps are visible, as we show in Chapter 15, but at least it is possible to see how these might be closed.

RECERTIFICATION

Recertification for doctors, although not for other members of the practice team, is now a live issue. There seems to be general acceptance of the principle that general practitioners should be able to show that they are keeping up to date and are effective in practice. The question is not so much whether as how to do this.[8-11]

When asked, most general practitioners seem to support recertification and accreditation. The principle was implicitly endorsed by two-thirds of general practitioners in 1992, when the General Medical Services Committee (GMSC) surveyed opinion in the profession.[12] A study in Cleveland revealed that 61% of respondents thought that recertification was necessary.[13] Most doctors favoured recertification at ten-year intervals. Clinical knowledge (82%), clinical skills (82%), prescribing practices (67%), standards of medical record keeping (60%) and consultation behaviour (58%) were the most popular subjects for scrutiny.

The GMSC proposal

The GMSC has published its own proposals.[14] The GMSC would like to see a five-yearly reappraisal based on a visit with the doctor. Subjects for discussion may include:

- practice documents, including the annual report
- the GP's participation in clinical audit, research and relevant activities
- videos of patient consultations
- a review of the practitioner's medical records.

The GMSC emphasizes that there would be no written examination. Similarly, because the process would be specific to the individual practitioner, there would be no assessment by proxy of the partners or of the function of the partnership as a whole. The premises would not be included, although the visitors may give advice.

In addition to the five-yearly assessment, the regional advisers in general practice or their representatives would conduct an annual review with a practitioner, which would include:

- assessing the previous year's educational activities
- reviewing the doctor's professional development during the previous year
- planning and approving the following year's educational activity.

The strength of the proposal is that it would extend the principle of external review to all doctors, albeit in the form of interviews. The main weakness is that it would rely heavily on the volume of documented educational experience – a difficulty because there is no clear linkage between taking part in educational events and performance.[15]

The RCGP is clearly interested in these developments. Fellowship by Assessment, a mid-career reassessment of a doctor's performance, is described in Chapter 15. It provides practical experience of review in action.

The GMC's contribution

The GMC can help in two ways. First, the recently published booklet *Good Medical Practice* gives doctors explicit guidance on their duties and responsibilities as registered practitioners.[16]

Second, the GMC now has powers to deal with persistently poor practice. Under new arrangements which start in 1997, the GMC will be able to assess a doctor's pattern of practice and, if the doctor's performance is thought to be so poor that patients are at risk, either to suspend the doctor from practice or restrict the doctor's registration until after retraining. General practitioners will normally be visited in their practices by assessors. The assessment will include an extended interview, an inspection of the clinical records and discussion with people who know about the doctor's work. There is also likely to be a written test of basic factual knowledge.

So, the GMC provides clear guidance about keeping up to date; protects the public from doctors who are not safe; and arranges retraining for doctors who fall behind.

LOOKING AHEAD

Recertification is coming – there seems to be general agreement about that. There are three general points to make.

First, general practitioners can now concentrate on their own professional development. The GMC will deal with poor practice. So the links with education can be strong. Recertification can be approached in a positive and constructive way.

Second, a way needs to be found of integrating recertification and practice accreditation. Perhaps complete practice accreditation should be expected to include duly certificated and recertificated practitioners.

Lastly, we cannot emphasize too strongly the link between the partnership and its responsibility for ensuring that each doctor in a practice performs well (Chapter 3). Prevention is better than cure.

REFERENCES

1 Royal College of General Practitioners (1994) *Quality and Audit in General Practice: Meanings and Definitions*. London: RCGP.

2 Bandaranayake R, Cameron D, Groseilliers J P *et al.* (1994) Maintenance of competence and/or re-certification: policy consideration. In *The*

Certification and Re-certification of Doctors (eds Newble D, Jolly B, Wakeford R). Cambridge: Cambridge University Press.

3   Lloyd J S (1979) Definitions of Competence in Specialties of Medicine. Chicago: American Board of Medical Specialties.

4   Rethans J J, Sturmans F, Drop R et al. (1991) Does competence of general practitioners predict their performance? Comparison between examination setting and actual practice. British Medical Journal; 303: 1377–80.

5   Irvine D H, Irvine S (1991) Making Sense of Audit. Oxford: Radcliffe Medical Press.

6   National Association of Health Authorities and Trusts (1994) Partners in Learning: Developing Postgraduate Training and Continuing Education for General Practice. London: NAHAT.

7   Ovretveit J (1992) Quality: an Introduction to Quality Method for Health Services. Oxford: Blackwell.

8   Gray D P (1992) Reaccrediting general practice. British Medical Journal; 305: 488–9.

9   Stanley I, Al-Sheri I (1993) Reaccreditation: the why, what and how. British Journal of General Practice; 43: 524–9.

10 Nichol F (1995) Making reaccreditation meaningful. British Journal of General Practice; 45: 321–4.

11 Richards T (1995) Recertifying general practitioners. British Medical Journal; 310: 1348–9.

12 General Medical Services Committee (1995) Interim report on individual reaccreditation: a discussion paper. Appendix in GMSC. Annual Report. London: BMA.

13 Sylvester S H H (1993) General practitioners' attitudes to professional reaccreditation. British Medical Journal; 307: 912-14.

14 General Medical Services Committee (1993) Task Group on Specialist Accreditation: a Discussion Paper. London: GMSC.

15 Burrows P (1995) Continuing medical education: a personal view. British Medical Journal; 310: 994.

16 General Medical Council (1995) Good Medical Practice. London: GMC.

15

External review in action

The proof of the pudding ...

Anon.

One of the nice things about general practice, and one of the benefits of its independent status, is that practices that have an outward-looking and exploratory approach to life can move on without having to wait for the results of national discussion, agreements and other bureaucratic processes to give them permission. This is particularly true today as there is debate as to whether, and in what form, recertification and practice accreditation shall be introduced. While this debate rolls on, a growing number of practices – often encouraged and supported financially by equally interested regional post-graduate organizations and health authorities – are helping to shape existing methods and approaches. They are finding out what works and what does not, what is acceptable to practices and what is not, and what should be changed and what should be kept. It reminds us very much of the early days of vocational training, when the leading teaching practices and schemes 'did their own thing', then shared their experiences. It was several years before the common ground became clear, around which the regulatory framework was then constructed.

We have given a full chapter to the stories of six practices that have had direct experience of one or other of the present-day approaches to external review, so that readers can acquire a 'hands-on' feel for what is involved, to be in a better position to judge for themselves whether they would like to try also. The common theme is of assessing performance against explicit operational and clinical standards that are either internal, external or more usually to be found in combination. All reviews are voluntary – no practice was required to undertake these exercises against its will. Some, such as Fellowship by Assessment of the RCGP, focus on the individual doctor and only to a lesser extent on the practice. Others, such as the British Standards Institution BS5750 (now properly called BS EN ISO 9000 because it is a European standard) and KFOA, are about specific areas of practice-based activity and therefore involve primarily the functioning of teams. We think the case histories illustrate, as no theoretical text can, just how interdependent are the questions of assessing the performance of individuals, the performance of practice teams and the practices as organizations to which all belong, because that is how general practice is. The sum is greater than the individual parts.

Of course, some will say that there is something special about these practices, that they are unrepresentative of general practice as a whole. This is true. But the key thing about them all, and our reason for choosing them, is that they show what can be done when some practices put their minds to it, and decide to demonstrate quality to the outside world.

In fact, the practices do present something of a cross-section of communities in Britain. They are by no means all in the 'leafy shires' popularly associated with easier practice conditions. On the contrary, two are in parts of the country where industry is in decline, unemployment is significant and there is a high index of social and health deprivation. Another is in the centre of London, with all the challenges that metropolitan practice presents.

We begin with the reaccreditation of a teaching practice, because teaching practice accreditation is the longest established approach to external review. It is the method which is best known and is well regarded and respected not only within general practice, but also by other specialties in medicine and by NHS management. General practice is proud of its teaching practice system, regarding it, rightly, as one of its greatest assets.

TEACHING PRACTICE ACCREDITATION

The accreditation of teaching practices has been in operation since vocational training was introduced in the early 1970s. It combines an assessment of the trainer and the practice by the regional post-graduate organization that is responsible for trainer appointments.[1]

The national standards required for training practices are set and published by the JCPTGP, and these carry RCGP endorsement for its membership examination. Each post-graduate organization uses these national standards as the basis for its own regional standards. Most regions have their own variations, which seek higher standards than the national norm on some aspects – rather as national clinical guidelines are adapted for local use. Over the years these national and regional standards have been progressively refined. At first they concentrated on the abilities of the doctor as a teacher and the general environment for learning furnished by the practice. Thus, there was a great deal of structure. Today, there is more emphasis on the ability of the doctor as a clinician as well as a teacher, and specific standards are set for the practice in areas such as medical records, prescribing and in the use of clinical audit. So now structural criteria tend to be taken for granted, with more emphasis on process aspects of quality and even, here and there, outcome.

The regional post-graduate organizations are themselves subject to periodic external peer review by the Joint Committee, to ensure that their processes of regional accreditation conform to the national requirements and standards, and work as intended. In the course of these visits, teaching practices are sampled by visitors, to ensure that they do indeed meet the necessary standards.

Case Study 36   Teaching practice accreditation

BACKGROUND TO PRACTICE

Lintonville Medical Group is a six-partner, teaching and fundholding practice in the north-east of England, in a former coal mining area with high unemployment and large pockets of severe deprivation within the community. The practice, formed in 1968, operates from the site of a former partner's home, and provides an excellent environment for the 14 000 patients who are registered with the practice, and for the 45 people who work there in addition to the partners.

WHY TEACHING?

The practice was founded in 1968, the year preceding the introduction of the first vocational training scheme for general practice in north-east England. The foundation partners decided that the new practice should be part of the scheme, partly because they believed in the ideas behind vocational training and wanted to support it and partly because they understood that involvement in teaching in future would expose the practice to external review, informally by the trainees who came to work at the practice and formally by the structured approach to trainer assessment which was then being developed by the local faculty of the RCGP and the people who were organizing the first training programmes.

The practice has chosen to retain its teaching status from that time to the present day. There have been several trainers. One became a course organizer for a short period before developing his research interests more fully, and another became regional adviser in general practice when these appointments were made.

Study Case 36: *continued*

WHO IS INVOLVED?

The practice has an explicit commitment to training. The designated trainer has lead responsibility for supervising the registrar and for implementing an agreed curriculum. Other partners and other staff are involved in teaching, which ensures that the registrar gains the widest possible perspective and benefits from the broad range of skills available in the practice.

At Lintonville the partnership takes ultimate responsibility for ensuring that training complies with the currently prevailing standards, and that the practice therefore continues to remain in good standing and maintain its teaching status. Current standards for teaching practices in the north of England involve not only the trainer but also the practice; thus, for example, there has to be a practice-wide commitment to clinical audit and the registrar is expected to be exposed to good prescribing and good record keeping, and must be able to learn about effective teamwork and practice management by seeing them done and by taking part.

Thus, the responsibility for training, which previously rested very much with the trainer, is today seen as a corporate practice responsibility delegated by the partnership to the trainer.

CURRENT METHOD OF ACCREDITATION

Teaching practice accreditation is for a fixed term, up to three years. Practices that are providing a good service with an experienced trainer can normally expect a three-year contract if all has gone well in the period of the previous contract.

The detailed method is similar to that which operates nationally, and which will therefore be familiar to any trainer. The 'official' review visit is undertaken by a team of three, the team comprising an associate adviser in general practice (the leader) and a representative each from the local medical committee and the North of England Faculty of the RCGP. Comprehensive documentation about both the trainer and the practice are completed beforehand, so that the visiting team not only has a good idea of what to expect, but is able to focus the visit on areas of particular interest or concern.

Study Case 36: *continued*

A final appearance before a university appointments committee was usual recently, but has now been dropped. The visiting panel has authority to renew the contract if all appears well and the new contract is likely to be fulfilled satisfactorily. The practice recognizes, however, that the university post-graduate organization reserves the right to ask for a full hearing if it is unsatisfied or has particular issues it wants to raise.

RESULTS

At the last visit the trainer and practice were asked to make some adjustments to their work as a condition of reaccreditation. The visitors recorded ways in which the trainer might take her professional development further, in particular by concentrating on her skills in clinical audit and practice management. The habit of building in 'improvements' in this way is usual, and has been found by the practice to focus discussion on areas where it should move forward.

BENEFITS

In a quarter-century of continuous involvement in teaching, the following are the main benefits which we feel may be attributed to this system of periodic reaccreditation.

- The practice has been stimulated to maintain its awareness of the outside world, and therefore how it compares and contrasts with other practices, and whether it is moving forwards or standing still.
- The review periods have provided the practice with an opportunity for internal stocktaking, which would in all honesty not have occurred with the same sense of urgency without the deadlines of reaccreditation and the prospect of outsiders looking in.
- The reviews have provided the trainers and the practice with regular opportunities to say what they think about the performance of the regional post-graduate organization, in particular where improvements could be made there. Thus, there is an element of mutual appraisal.
- Overall, the idea of external review has been found to be so helpful that, in recent years, the decision was taken by the partners to explore this further. In particular, the practice became a first-wave fundholder primarily because of the opportunities it saw there for developing itself as a provider, working to outside 'contracted'

Case Study 36: *continued*

standards. Even more recently, the practice successfully completed the GPQA version of BS EN ISO 9000 to provide more focus on the quality of the organization. Its GPQA status is being maintained through six-monthly visits. And two partners are keen to undergo Fellowship by Assessment (FBA) of the RCGP as soon as they become eligible.

- As the system of periodic reaccreditation for teaching continues to evolve, there is now far more emphasis on the personal professional development of the trainer. This interactive approach between trainer, practice and post-graduate organization is helpful and constructive, not least because of the practical support given by the region to trainer development.

PROBLEMS

There are the anxieties that go with preparing for and completing accreditation successfully, but that sort of anxiety is part of the process! Specific weaknesses have been identified from time to time, almost all invariably known to the practice beforehand but of the kind 'we had not quite got round to fixing it'. Completed summaries of case notes and, at one stage, a decidedly shaky repeat prescribing system are good examples.

COSTS

Reaccreditation visits, including the pre-review visits by an associate adviser, are paid for by the post-graduate organization.

The time and effort spent by the practice on preparation is absorbed into the overall costs of teaching, which have to be set against the trainer's grant and the contribution the registrar makes to the work of the practice.

COMMENTARY

Involvement in training practice accreditation has provided the trainer and the practice with regular opportunities for stocktaking and review, and for making adjustments where these are thought necessary.

Case Study 36: *continued*

Accreditation has always seemed to be an endorsement, by independent people, of what the practice itself wants to do. So the primary initiative has always lain with the practice. But, being human, the practice would be the first to recognize that its good intentions can often exceed its ability to deliver; reaccreditation can be a timely reminder of that and a stimulus to close the gap.

Sarah Cleverly, trainer and chair of the partnership, Lintonville Medical Group, Ashington, Northumberland

RCGP FELLOWSHIP BY ASSESSMENT

The traditional route to fellowship of the RCGP[2] by nomination of existing fellows served the College well in its earlier years, but the expanding membership created its own problems. In particular, the process tended to exclude excellent general practitioners who delivered high-quality care yet were not involved in College work or in teaching or research.

Building on the College's Quality Initiative of 1983 and the system of practice assessments introduced at that time, known as 'What Sort of Doctor', the College developed the concept of a second route to fellowship through the demonstration of high-quality care to patients.[3] It was envisaged that such a process would require the definition of quality care, the evolution of standards, and a peer review system both to ensure the standards were met and to exploit the potential.

After extensive pilot work, the first version of FBA was introduced in 1988. The 60 criteria of quality have been evolving since then by a process of annual review, but the principles remain: any College member of five years standing who feels that he or she can demonstrate high standards in all areas specified (no criterion can be failed) is eligible for FBA. A member's achievement of the standards is demonstrated through a written submission. The practice is then visited by three fellows of the College for three days. As with other accreditation methods, there is extensive documentation aimed at revealing both individual performance as a clinician and the performance of the practice as an organization. So, for instance, the practitioner will be asked to furnish the assessors with videotapes of consultations as well as details of clinical guidelines in use, the results of clinical audit against these, and so on.

The gestation for FBA as an alternative route to fellowship of the College was lengthy, but it was finally approved by the RCGP Council in May 1989.[3]

Case Study 37   Fellowship by Assessment (FBA)

BACKGROUND TO THE PRACTICE

The Collingham Practice is a rural dispensing practice serving over 5500 patients. The medical centre is partner owned. The practice is fundholding and teaches vocational registrars and undergraduate students. The partnership consists of four medical partners and the practice manager, called the executive partner. The practice has an extensive system of clinical audit, management and general staff meetings, in all of which the chairmanship rotates around all the members, with a chairmanship rota published in advance.

DECISION-MAKING PROCESS

The main motivation to do FBA was twofold: we felt that we were practising to a very high standard and we welcomed a chance for that to be recognized; and we wanted to be among the first applicants. The practice had, and continues to have, a strong innovatory streak.

Three of the four partners in the practice were eligible (one was not a member of the College at the time) and we reviewed all the criteria involved in FBA together. There were no structural problems: the focus was on *demonstrating*, through a formidable documentation task, that we met the standard of FBA.

METHODS USED

The work was divided among the entire practice. Some criteria refer to the practice itself, for example meeting the criteria regarding the practice's policy on continuity of care necessitated an audit to demonstrate that continuity was effective. In this case one of the three applicants volunteered to write the policy, another drew up the plan of audit and one of the receptionists was recruited to carry out the audit. The resulting material was incorporated into all three applications.

Many criteria refer to the personal work of the applicant and we each had to do our own work for this. But we were able to learn from each other and offer advice and support. The receptionists became skilled at responding to one doctor's request by producing the equivalent medical records for the others.

Case Study 37: *continued*

Applicants usually take some time to prepare for FBA; we did so in only two months.

ACCREDITATION PROCESS

The first partner was visited on a very hot day in July, with the other two visited a week later. The time from first decision to assessment visit was therefore just over two months – a tribute to both the existing standards in the practice and the commitment of the staff. The visits caused anxiety and enjoyment at the same time.

BENEFITS

The cohesion of the team was tested to its limit, and was found not only to be strong but to be strengthened by effort. Although we had surveyed our care, the process revealed many deficiencies. We all realized that measuring was one thing, improving was another. This discussion was vital for the practice.

The culture that facilitated FBA was one that helped us cope with the health service reforms, and we have since entered fundholding without undue trauma.

Medical audit

There was a renewed commitment to conventional medical audit. Before starting on FBA we already had a limited number of written protocols. For FBA we quickly agreed a further set of clinical guidelines and 'audited' them in some haste – we asked receptionists to pull notes and someone (often the doctors, sometimes senior receptionists or secretaries) gathered the data. After FBA we reviewed each guideline and did what we should have done the first time: we compared our policies with the literature and argued the case for each criterion until we could justify them to ourselves and any outside body. We studied the care outlined in our applications for FBA and identified those areas that we regarded as unsatisfactory. After a while we repeated the surveys, converting our efforts into *real* audits, and we looked for evidence of improvement.

Our clinical guidelines are drawn together into a booklet that contains over 25 agreed sets. If a visitor, patient or registrar wishes to

Case Study 37: *continued*

see the standards that we set ourselves and the extent to which we meet them, the guidelines and their audits are available; indeed, many of the latter are published in our annual report. In more recent years the practice and community nurses have become more involved in agreeing protocols and the practice employs a data analyst, one of whose tasks is to ensure that the data gathering part of clinical audit does in fact occur.

Case-based auditing

The next benefit that came from FBA was the notion of case-based auditing. One FBA criterion had asked each of us to report on the 'presentation' to 'management' of a group of our patients with a major diagnosis, especially cancer. In our monthly lunchtime significant event meetings we discuss individual patients who have experienced an important clinical or administrative event. For example we write down every new myocardial infarction, stroke or cancer diagnosis, every visit to an asthmatic, diabetic or epileptic patient presenting with an acute episode and every unplanned pregnancy or suicide attempt. In addition, we note down every patient complaint, prescribing error, unavailability of appointments or staff crisis.

All nurses, managers and doctors are invited to significant event audit meetings and there are only two simple rules: total confidentiality and avoidance of blame. If someone has mismanaged a patient or situation, it is the practice's responsibility to ensure that it does not happen again. Everyone chooses a case from their list and briefly describes it. The others then ask questions to ensure that all the lessons are learnt. Where appropriate, clinical guidelines are the yardstick against which our care is judged. When they do not cover the area, the same principles apply – we discuss and agree a consensus view of 'best care' and then apply it to the case being discussed.

As a result of this process we celebrate good care. This happens all too seldom in primary care; we take excellence for granted and concentrate on mistakes. In significant event auditing we may hear about a nurse who took a blood test from a 'tired' patient and diagnosed leukaemia, or of a patient complaint handled well, with the situation defused. The amount of behavioural and structural change is far greater after a case-based discussion than after discussing the results of a conventional audit. While the latter appeals to the head, a

Case Study 37: *continued*

significant event appeals to the heart – and change is an emotional process.

DIFFICULTIES ENCOUNTERED

Time

For us FBA represented a spirit of work – a spirit of the time – that halted all other non-clinical work for three months. For others, the work and disruption can be spread out, but it is still considerable.

Perhaps our greatest difficulty was that of being trail blazers. We had no 'expert' to answer our queries, and no case law to fall back on. This created uncertainty; thankfully, we were too busy to allow this to distract us.

COMMENT

The greatest lesson for me was that succeeding in the very difficult is a spur to tackle the 'impossible'. Our short period of self-congratulation and complacency was cut short by an awareness of the need to maintain and renew our momentum. We may not have been able to verbalize the post-FBA test, the 'impossible task', but it can now be seen to be the achievement of a cultural shift. The extent to which we have succeeded can only be judged in the future, and I feel that we have been only partially successful so far.

The second major lesson is that the FBA criteria contained the points that we had to learn. Although those relating to audit were very rudimentary and have now been radically improved, we could meet the letter of the criteria without really complying with the spirit: we could audit but we did not necessarily improve. So the greatest long-term effect of the FBA has been, in my judgement, its catalytic effect on our quality assurance programme; indeed, it stimulated the programme itself. While we must still strive to avoid complacency, we have come further than I ever dreamt might be possible down the path towards having a quality culture – a state in which as many opportunities as possible are taken to improve care.

The advent of real guidelines, agreed and adhered to not because of an external imperative, such as FBA, but because we believed that they represented good care, was a real gain, and it continues to

Case Study 37: *continued*

underpin our clinical care. Many doctors complain that clinical guidelines inhibit them and are unnecessarily bureaucratic. That is, however, to confuse the freedom to perform bad medicine with the responsibility to define and attempt one's best. The latter requires a voluntary surrender of the right to treat patients less well for a common definition of 'good care'.

The arrival of significant event auditing has given a new dimension to our quality assurance. Fellowship by Assessment was the time when we had the courage to declare our quality to the world outside the practice. It was a seminal moment which might have led to different outcomes; it has, in fact, resulted in greater commitment to a quality culture – to quality assurance being part of everyday practice. The work and sweat involved in FBA has, I believe, been amply justified.

The rush from decision to application was such that we did not have time or opportunity to reflect too deeply on the process or its possible effects. There was a collective buzz from the team working well towards a shared goal, and a sense of achievement because our previous changes were now bearing fruit.

Mike Pringle, general practitioner, Collingham Practice, Nottinghamshire

BRITISH STANDARDS INSTITUTION BS 5750/ BS EN ISO 9000

The British Standards Institution (BSI) offers accreditation to a practice by assessing whether it has a quality system that the Institution can register. BS EN ISO 9000 is a familiar international quality standard that enables organizations to establish, document and maintain a proper quality management system. Its origins lie in manufacturing, where mistakes can be costly. It has formed the basis of a great number of the quality management systems and certification schemes in the UK. Over 25 000 UK firms now have accreditation.

General Practice Quality Assured is one of a number of routes to achieving BS EN ISO 9000. It was developed by the Medical Protection Society, which believes that a clearly identified mark of achievement will provide a focus for improvement in practice management and, over time, a well-recognized sign of commitment to delivering effective patient services. At the core of GPQA is the belief that the root of most organizational problems in general practice is a lack of agreed procedures which, if they were sound and in place, could be used as a tool for improving performance and communication. It is a means of confirming and testing quality standards.

The BSI approach lays down guidelines and criteria for a quality system based on the principles of the quality loop – akin to the quality management cycle – in which the practice determines its own criteria and standards of good practice. The test for accreditation is whether the practice implements its own standards thoroughly and consistently. The final inspection is carried out by a person appointed by the BSI, who makes a thorough inspection on site.

British Standards Institution accreditation involves a considerable amount of documentation and effort on the part of the practice team. Its supporters like in particular the freedom it gives a practice to set its own standards. However, there are critics who believe that the process is unnecessarily bureaucratic and expensive for what it does. Practices need to bear these pros and cons in mind when making their choice. Interestingly, the practice in our case study (and the practice in Case Study 36) succeeded in keeping the paperwork under control, so making the procedure quite acceptable to it.

Case Study 38   BSI/GPQA

BACKGROUND TO THE PRACTICE

The Grove Health Centre serves some 12 000 patients with a full complement of clinical, managerial, secretarial and receptionist staff, and has attached staff including health visitors, district nurses, chiropodist, HIV/AIDS counsellor and dietitian. The practice is housed in a purpose-built health centre. All day-to-day operational matters are managed by the practice manager and senior members of the staff. The doctors meet monthly with the practice manager to deal with policy issues and the senior partner acts as chairman.

WHY THE PRACTICE DECIDED TO GO FOR GPQA

Like many other service sector organizations, the practice had begun to think about quality and how to test its standards against external criteria. More specifically the decision to choose GPQA was taken in order:

• **to gain confidence in our own systems and procedures**
• **to demonstrate a serious commitment to quality**
• **to remove waste and duplication**

Case Study 38: *continued*

- to reinforce our reputation locally, to patients
- to improve the collection and use of data
- to impress suppliers and suppliers of resources, e.g. the local FHSA
- to use it as a management tool
- to identify training needs
- to seek third party approval – audit and accreditation process.

THE DECISION-MAKING PROCESS

The decision to embark on GPQA was made by the partners and practice manager. The practice manager was appointed quality representative and had overall responsibility for the training and implementation programme. One of the partners acted as the GP representative and undertook to train as an internal auditor. A meeting was held with the staff to explain the scheme and to secure their support.

WHO WAS INVOLVED?

The practice manager and the senior partner were involved in preparing the original GPQA guidelines. Once these were launched the practice manager worked closely with the 'quality partner' to design and implement the system. The key to successful implementation was the involvement of all the staff in drafting procedures, leaving the manager to structure the procedures to comply with the requirements of good procedural practice.

PROCESS INVOLVED

Quality clubs

Training a practice to receive GPQA is achieved through quality clubs, which bring together a number of general practitioners and practice managers for 12 sessions. At the training sessions we were guided through preparing the system and writing quality manuals and procedures. After each session we went away to work with our own staff, with a trainer who was available on the telephone to help with day-to-day queries. The participants got to know each other and created a self-help group, exchanging ideas and sharing common procedures.

As part of the quality club arrangements the practice manager and a partner attended a one-day audit training session. Auditing for GPQA is about watching people perform tasks in a specific procedure and

Case Study 38: *continued*

informally interviewing them to ensure that they have been adequately trained for the work they are undertaking. It also provides an opportunity to review each procedure and for the staff to suggest changes.

Where there is a clear discrepancy between what should be happening and what actually happens the auditor raises a *corrective action form*. This provides for a formal system which ensures that a discrepancy has been recognized and that agreed action is completed by the member of staff responsible.

The quality manual

The first stage of the process towards accreditation is the publication of a *quality manual*. This document describes how the practice meets the GPQA standard. Although it is used by the assessors as the basis for their assessment, it is also a public statement of the practice's values and may be made available to patients as well as other health agencies and suppliers.

The manual includes a *history of the practice* and the *purpose/ scope* of the manual. It has a *policy statement*, drafted by the partners, confirming the practice's commitment to quality and the practice's overall objectives or 'mission' of the practice. This is supported by a description of the practice's organization and the roles and responsibilities of key personnel.

Management review is a method that ensures that the system is regularly reviewed and updated. The terms of reference of management review form an integral part of the quality manual. We decided to set up a management review group comprising representatives of the whole of the practice. The group meets quarterly to review the system and authorize changes, where necessary.

Contract review or provision of services describes the agreements in place with the local community trust and FHSA. It is also a requirement that pertinent copies of the general practice terms of service are held by the quality representative. A system for receiving feedback from patients must also be included in this section.

Document control is another important aspect of the standard. This ensures that all documents and forms within the system are kept up to date and renewed when necessary. Purchasing is also kept under

Case Study 38: *continued*

control by ensuring that a purchasing procedure is in place and that products are only purchased from approved suppliers.

The final section of the quality manual refers to training. It is a requirement that the practice is able to demonstrate a commitment to identify training needs and provide the training and resources to meet them.

Process control

General Practice Quality Assured includes specific requirements for process control. These are basic general practice procedures which must be in place before assessment. They include:

- a clearly defined appointment system that differentiates between urgent and non-urgent cases
- a home visiting service that discriminates between emergency, urgent and non-urgent cases
- a documented system for dealing with out-of-hours calls
- agreed guidelines for referrals to other agencies
- a system for dealing with repeat prescriptions
- a system for ensuring that patients whose test results indicate a serious abnormality are contacted by the doctor.

While GPQA does not include clinical work, there are a number of requirements of the medical personnel. These include the inspection of drugs, medical dressings and appliances, ensuring that they use equipment that has been calibrated and segregating products deemed to be damaged or passed their expiry date.

Opportunity to improve

This is a new procedure born out of GPQA for the practice called *opportunity to improve*. This enables any member of the team to make suggestions on improving quality or highlighting trends when things go wrong. Once raised there is a commitment by the quality representative to ensure that a response is given or an explanation as to why a procedure cannot be changed.

Internal quality audits are a mechanism for ensuring that each procedure is audited within the organization at least once a year. This

Case Study 38: *continued*

has involved training the practice manager and lead partner in how to complete audits and to introduce an audit plan into the practice.

Procedures

After the quality manual was produced, the next phase was to ensure that the system was running according to the indicators in the manual. Our approach was to ask each section within the practice to write its own procedure documents. These documents highlight the key quality issues throughout the practice including the following:

- key reception procedures, e.g. registering new patients, making appointments, taking messages
- information management, e.g. maintenance of the computer system, data entry, dealing with FHSA claim forms
- secretarial procedures, e.g. referrals, management of petty cash, dealing with insurance reports
- nursing procedures, e.g. ensuring drugs are within their expiry dates, checking refrigerator temperatures, monitoring cervical smear results.

Once the staff had submitted their work to the practice manager, he drafted the procedures into a consistent format, before formally introducing each of them as quality documents.

THE ACCREDITATION PROCESS

Preassessment visit

The last of the quality club days takes place in the practice before the assessment visit. All the trainers at the quality club have experience of assessing firms for registration for BS EN ISO 9000 so it gave us a good 'dress rehearsal' for the real thing. It also provided an opportunity to fine tune some of our procedures.

The assessment visit

For a practice of our size the visit lasted one day. The visit opened with a meeting with the partners and manager to formulate a programme for the day. Throughout the day the assessor interviewed a number of the staff and watched a number of activities. Although the assessor may not have detailed knowledge of how a practice operates the assessment is designed in such a way that the assessor is able to pick up any

Case Study 38: *continued*

procedure and check if it is happening in accordance with the protocol. Detailed knowledge is not necessary. It is the quality representative's role to accompany the assessor and explain the various
activities in broad terms, if necessary. After preparing a detailed report
the assessor returns to the meeting to make a recommendation. In our
case it was to receive certification. The day ended with us opening a
well-deserved bottle of champagne!

OBSTACLES

Time

The registration process for GPQA is time-consuming. The practice
manager was released for 12 quality club days, plus 24 days to write,
modify and present procedures. The amount of doctor time required is
minimal, involving one day audit training and about one and a half
days for auditing in the practice. A good secretary is essential for producing the documentation.

Management of change

As in any new system communication was a vital component of the
change. To assist this the practice manager produced a regular
newsletter entitled *Towards BS EN ISO 9000*, which gave all members
of the team regular updates on the process towards accreditation.

Costs

Direct costs
GPQA itself costs £4000 including full training and the initial assessment. In addition, a large practice can expect to pay £200 a year for its
calibration programme. This is used to ensure that all equipment in the
practice used for accurate measurement, such as sphygmomanometers
(biannually), weighing scales (annually) and the practice autoclave
(quarterly), are calibrated and serviced on a regular basis.

Indirect costs
The most significant indirect cost is the staff time to develop the
system and once in place to service it. Apart from the time costs of
the above, once certification is obtained, the management representative can expect to spend two to three hours a week on the system,
with up to two hours per month thereafter.

Case Study 38: *continued*

Standards

GPQA provides a number of guidelines that help practices achieve the BSI kitemark, but there are no specific standards laid down externally. The standards are generated internally in the practice. The assessor is looking for explicit standards, not making judgements about them.

Organizational commitment

The managers of the practice have to be absolutely committed to the process. It requires an investment in both time and finance.

BENEFITS

We benefited in particular from the following.

- **The identification of exactly and explicitly how things are done in the practice: in exploring and formalizing activities, opportunities were created to improve and refine existing practices.**
- **The application process developed a sense of teamwork among the partners and staff. All the staff had an opportunity to participate in various degrees according to their own abilities and motivation.**
- **Knowledge was shared among the practice staff in a way which did not happen before. New members of staff can come into the practice and quickly familiarize themselves with documentation designed to brief them before they start work.**
- **Patients had opportunities to make comments on the services by either completing a suggestion slip or making more serious complaints through an in-house complaints procedure.**

COMMENT

BS EN ISO 9000 is somewhat bureaucratic and top-heavy with written procedures and documentation, but the assessors are more interested in seeing that 'what you say you do, you do' than trawling through volumes of procedures. Documentation can be kept to a minimum, and as part of our ongoing management review we are constantly seeking ways to cut down on the paperwork and reduce the number of procedures.

BS EN ISO 9000 was aimed at manufacturing processes, and many of the component parts of the standard are not a prime concern for GP surgeries which have limited purchasing requirements and inspection

Case Study 38: *continued*

and test criteria. General Practice Quality Assured has made a useful attempt to make the standard relevant to general practice, and no doubt more refining will be achieved as more practices become interested.

The concept of quality clubs is an important feature of GPQA, and my advice to any practice embarking on either GPQA or alternative routes to BS EN ISO 9000 is to make the most out of sharing experiences with other practices.

General Practice Quality Assured is primarily aimed at large practices but it is as relevant to a small single-handed practice as it is to a large fundholding practice. In industry a BS EN ISO 9000 logo will be appearing on the vehicles of a sole trading car mechanic or a multinational company. We put ours on our practice notepaper!

Renos Pittarides, practice manager, Grove Health Centre, West London

KING'S FUND ORGANISATIONAL AUDIT

King's Fund Organisational Audit is a national approach to setting and monitoring standards for providers of health services. In 1993 the King's Fund extended the audit it carries out in hospitals to general practices.[4]

The method differs significantly from BS EN ISO 9000 in that the King's Fund itself publishes standards covering most aspects of the organization of work and of the environment for care within general practice. The standards are concerned with the systems and structures that the King's Fund believes should be in place to support high-quality patient care. The standards are designed to reflect patients' expectations of quality care and to represent a consensus on currently accepted professional practice. They cover areas which include the management arrangements of a practice, contracts, communications, practice procedures and protocols, patient access, buildings and equipment, arrangements for audit, and so on.

Practices applying for assessment first arm themselves with the standards, and then work towards their implementation. The King's Fund offers a consultancy service to help practices achieve the standards. There are two workshops and a presurvey visit before the survey itself, which lasts one and a half days. When the practice is ready, it is then subject to inspection by a trained team consisting of a general practitioner, practice manager and another external manager (often from an FHSA), to verify that the standards are in fact being observed.

The charges for King's Fund audit vary between £5700 and £7200 (+VAT) depending on practice size and numbers of staff involved. Currently all are sponsored by FHSA and health boards. Seventy-one practices will undergo King's Fund audit in 1996.

Case Study 39   The King's Fund Organisational Audit (KFOA)

BACKGROUND TO THE PRACTICE

This is a first-wave fundholding and training practice serving 17 500 patients with a full complement of attached and ancillary staff. It is housed in a ten-year-old purpose-built surgery. A board of directors of all the partners manages the practice, with the help of a practice business and development manager. This manager has delegated powers of authority and responsibility for the day-to-day management of the practice.

WHY KING'S FUND ORGANISATIONAL AUDIT?

The practice accepted an invitation in 1991 to be one of the nine pilot sites selected in England, Wales and Northern Ireland to take the KFOA approach into a primary care setting. Before this, the practice had been reviewing the next steps as regards initiatives on quality assurance, based on its belief that the quality of patient care depends on good clinical practice and, as importantly, on good management, organization and delivery of patient services.

The specific reasons for launching on this project were as follows.

- It was relevant to the practice's organizational and professional development, which was concerned with developing and testing specific standards and criteria in a primary care setting.
- The Organisational Audit fitted the practice's philosophy of skill and knowledge combined with care and teaching.
- It provided a chance to bridge the secondary/primary interface.
- As the local hospital unit was first on the KFOA acute programme, the exercise was felt to be important because one of the reasons the practice proceeded with first-wave fundholding was to support and to contribute to the development of the local hospital services for the benefit of the local community.
- It offered a team approach to audit.

Case Study 39: *continued*

- The King's Fund itself has credibility and respect as a body that seeks to stimulate good practice and innovations in all aspects of health care.
- The FHSA and district health authority (DHA) were willing to support the initiative in terms of finance and time, to promote even closer working relationships.
- The invitation was viewed as another opportunity to participate in a 'first', and one which would complement the first year of the fund-holding initiative.

THE DECISION-MAKING PROCESS

The decision to go ahead with the application was taken by the partners, the manager and the practice nurse team leader. The consultation process included external consultation with the chairman of the local DHA and the chief executive of the FHSA. Inside the practice the consultation and communication processes were both structured via the weekly primary health care meetings and weekly practice meetings and regular practice nurse meetings. Nearer the time of the survey the process was enhanced by a television series on the KFOA acute programme taking place in London.

WHO WAS INVOLVED?

All members of the primary health care team together with the stakeholders (FHSA and DHA managers) participated. The subsequent work was coordinated by the steering group, with the practice business and development manager and the practice nurse team facilitator nominated as the survey coordinators responsible for the presurvey documentation. The steering group was made up of 'volunteers' from each of the different professional groups working within the surgery.

METHOD OF WORKING

The steering group had two complementary tasks:

1 to draft criteria/standards for the key areas of nursing and management within primary care
2 to undertake the responsibility of testing all the standards being developed by the pilot sites.

Case Study 39: *continued*

It was then charged with sharing, communicating, educating and preparing the practice and the team for the implementation of the criteria and the survey.

Having contributed to the development of the standards and criteria, the steering group then planned for the successful delivery of the second task, namely to implement the KFOA process in the practice. It was decided at the start to utilize the existing channels of communication rather than set up new ones, and therefore the weekly primary health care team meetings provided the valuable forum for progress reports.

Communication and education became the main focus for the work. The newsletter and patient participation group proved most valuable, especially when completing the presurvey questionnaires from the College of Health. The practice completed presurvey documentation about the practice (including practice leaflets and practice reports), the proposed timetable and the baseline audit. It is this baseline, undertaken by the practice, which forms the framework for the surveyors. It is the practice's view of where they are implementing the criteria and standards, and identifies priorities for action.

The baseline audit provided the key areas for improvement; the whole team worked in earnest for the survey. All stakeholders were kept up to date, culminating in a specially designed 'learning for change' course for the partners and myself the weekend before the survey.

The survey was undertaken by an independent team of three senior health professionals chosen for their experience, knowledge, credibility and appropriateness for the organization being surveyed. The team included a general practitioner, a practice manager and a manager working for a community trust. The role of the surveyors was to assess compliance with the standards, to commend good practice and to recommend improvements.

The first day of the survey included a review of the external channels of communication, for example interviews with representatives from the FHSA, acute and community trusts and the Community Health Council (CHC). The surveyors worked in the practice for two days, reviewing documentation, interviewing key players, and meeting as many of the primary health care team as possible within the timetable. The debriefing involved the partners, practice manager and other key players. A detailed written report followed six weeks later.

Case Study 39: *continued*

COSTS

The direct costs of £5000 payable to the King's Fund were financed by matched funding from the practice and the FHSA and DHA.

The indirect costs were mainly those relating to the time spent by all members of the primary health care team, particularly the secretarial and administrative support and the management and nursing personnel, in enabling the whole project to get off the ground. Time was also spent on training and on 'away days', steering group and progress meetings. Printing, postage and stationery added to the running costs, which were approximately £7000 for the whole of the two-year pilot phase. The running costs of the established programme are much less.

RESULTS

There was a striking improvement of 80% achievement of compliance with the standards at the survey time averaged over all standards, compared with a 47% compliance at the baseline audit stage the previous year.

BENEFITS

The primary health care team has not only contributed to the development of standards against which actual performance can be measured in a primary care facility but also tested the standards rigorously and volunteered the practice for assessment. Such an assessment made this practice the first to undergo survey in the King's Fund programme. The external team of surveyors highlighted good practice and gave recommendations for future improvement. Above all, the exercise is remembered as true teamwork in action, a feeling which continues. The practice is committed to reassessment by the King's Fund in 1995.

The process enabled us to continue to improve organizationally and professionally, and many new opportunities in teamworking and education have arisen by adopting a continuous improvement programme. These have included the setting up of in-house multidisciplinary and interprofessional education programmes, with post-graduate education approval, to address quality improvements and standards

Case Study 39: *continued*

specifically to the professions allied to medicine, including chiropody, dietetics and physiotherapy.

Unexpected internal learning opportunities have arisen through the King's Fund with their organization of surveyor training and seminars on quality improvement in primary health care.

Teamworking with members serving in the local community has been beneficial when developing a Primary Care Charter, effective Health of the Nation objectives and a new Teen Screen drop-in clinic. Networking too with other pilot sites has brought the added value of shared good practice and friendship.

As a pilot site we experienced the added opportunity of moving from the project stage to the full-blown programme, and as such enjoy the new slimline user-friendly manual in which the standards are weighted to help teams prioritize the work. They fall into the three categories of essential, good and desirable practice.

In addition the following benefits accrued:

- an explicit and public demonstration of our commitment to quality assurance and to continuous improvement
- improved patient care by providing a framework for the continuous review of the systems and processes which must be in place for the provision of effective and efficient health care services
- the ability to demonstrate good practice, and the ability to rise to challenges
- training to specific standards, e.g. the nursing team working together on wound care and the development of joint protocols, standards and care management plans
- the ability to demonstrate the organizational fitness of the practice to undertake new initiatives, such as our application to become a practice nurse training practice, and to continue to easily satisfy existing assessments such as the premises and facilities review by the FHSA
- organizational fitness, from which other quality developments can flow, such as more sophisticated clinical audit and Investors in People.

Case Study 39: *continued*

UNEXPECTED PROBLEMS ON THE WAY

With any new initiative there is always suspicion of change, and often mistrust. Through our own poor communication, some professional groups in the practice at first thought the partners and the manager were trying to impose standards on their professions. This was particularly evident when trying to work with social services and some professions allied to medicine.

Despite our intention to complete the work at our local community hospital, which was also undergoing KFOA, there was disappointingly slow progress on joint standard setting with the local hospital team.

The resource issues of people, time, space and finance had to be finely balanced with the priorities in the practice. The paperwork could have got on top of us if we had not set up a way of managing it effectively and quickly introduced a King's Fund resource in the practice library which could be accessed by all the team and kept up to date easily.

COMMENTARY

This audit process is an approach that has won on-going commitment to quality assurance in the practice. Like many other practices, we had never planned far enough ahead to be an effective organization. It has also been one way of keeping the practice up to date within and outwith the health care business environment – locally, regionally, nationally and internationally.

To participate in the programme demands a flexible and new approach to work practices, and the programme itself was a valuable resource that promoted joint learning and encouraged the work of quality improvement groups within the practice looking at, for example, access/appointment review and patient information.

It is around the external standards offered that the organizational fitness of a practice and its extended team can be measured, assessed and developed to provide optimum patient care. It facilitates the management challenge of questioning whether things could be done better or in a different way.

While this organizational audit does not specifically measure the personal or professional fitness of the members of the team, it does

Case Study 39: *continued*

provide the framework to help us address other quality initiatives, such as the Investors in People award and Fellowship by Assessment. We propose to do that.

Sandra E A Gower, practice business and development manager, Bennetts End Surgery, Hertfordshire

INVESTORS IN PEOPLE

The Investors in People award is a nationally recognized standard of excellence devised by industry leaders for training and developing all employees to achieve the objectives set out in the business plan of the organization. It aims to improve the performance of an organization by releasing the full potential of its workforce. It attempts to ensure that the needs of an organization – whatever its size or type – are matched by the skills and motivation of its staff.

There are four main parts: commitment, planning, action and evaluation. Each part has a number of assessment indicators (24 in total) used by the Training and Enterprise Council (TEC) to decide whether the organization has met the Investors in People standard. The practice must be able to demonstrate that it meets every indicator by allowing randomly selected staff to be interviewed and by offering supporting documentary evidence.

Case Study 40   Investors in People award

BACKGROUND TO THE PRACTICE

The practice is an eight-partner training practice serving 20 000 patients and supported by a full complement of attached staff and 24 employed staff. We operate from a health authority-owned purpose-built health centre in a semiurban area. The practice is substantially involved with research and audit, one partner being a member of the local Medical Audit Advisory Group (MAAG). The management structure of the practice includes an executive partner who works with the practice manager, reporting to monthly partnership meetings. There is a chair who is elected on a three-year term alongside the executive partner.

Case Study 40: *continued*

WHY THE PRACTICE DECIDED TO APPLY FOR THE INVESTORS IN PEOPLE AWARD

In 1992 the practice heard about the Investors in People award and realized that it corresponded to the staff training and development requirements of the practice. By working towards these standards and achieving the award we felt that we would give the staff the recognition they deserved for their efforts during the previous few years when there had been much instability and change in the practice. We were also keen to assess practice progress against an extremely rigorous external standard, and had attended seminars to compare some other methods, such as BS EN ISO 9000. We felt we should develop the people in the practice first, before looking at systems.

It was important to obtain a public commitment from the partners, leading from the front. The implications in terms of time, costs and benefits were discussed at partnership meetings before sending a letter to the TEC declaring our commitment.

METHOD OF WORKING

The TEC provided the Investor in People toolkit. This involved conducting a staff and management survey, to ascertain how the practice measured up to the standard set.

The survey

The survey comprised a list of questions to which the answer was 'yes', 'no' or 'don't know'. We then compared the management view of the practice with the staff view, which showed up differences of perception.

We analysed the results of these two surveys and discovered that many questions had a low percentage of 'yes' answers. We aimed to increase the number of 'yes' answers to 80% (some were standing at 20%) for each question, and then we would be able to apply for assessment.

Action plan

Using this information we produced an action plan, showing what we had to do and how we intended to do it, in order to satisfy all the assessment indicators.

Case Study 40: *continued*

The action plan had two main parts:

1 the development of service standards
2 the development of people.

Service standards
At a staff meeting we set about defining service standards by producing a comprehensive list of services provided to internal customers (each other) and external customers (patients, FHSA suppliers, etc.). Having agreed the service standards throughout the practice, we built in monitoring systems and encouraged staff groups to review performance at their monthly meetings.

We then looked at any interface issues between groups, e.g. reception and the treatment room appointments. Agreements were reached and guidelines and protocols were produced.

Staff development
Alongside the development of service standards we set about further staff development. We used the job descriptions to create a list of skills, knowledge and attributes for each role in the practice, including the partners' skills matrix. This information was then used in the appraisal system by both the appraisee (to self-assess) before the interview and during the interview as a measure against the requirements of the role. This assisted in drawing up a personal development plan for everyone in the practice, including training and skills already obtained (to identify underutilized skills) and those requiring further development.

For the first time the partners were included in the appraisal system. The practice manager was responsible for conducting the appraisals and therefore clinical aspects of the work were not included. All this was done on a voluntary basis. Each partner took part, with the executive partner leading the way.

From the appraisals and further staff and partner surveys a training plan for the practice was drawn up showing topics to be covered and objectives to be met. From this training plan a programme showing dates and times of training events was created.

The evaluation

At this point we were well on the way to satisfying the first three parts of the award: commitment, planning and action. The final part of the

Case Study 40: *continued*

evaluation is widely accepted as the most difficult part to satisfy. It is divided into assessment indicators to show that:

- the investment, the competence and commitment of employees and the use made of skills learned are reviewed at all levels against the practice's objectives and targets
- the effectiveness of training and development is reviewed at the top level and leads to renewed commitment and target setting.

A training assessment form was introduced which asks questions of the participants at three stages.

1 before the training: what do you hope to get out of this training?
2 immediately after the training: what did you learn and how will you put this into practice?
3 three months later: are you still using the learning in practice and, if not, why not?

These forms were then analysed to assess the benefits and quality of each training event.

At subsequent appraisals this information was used to assess individuals' progress towards both personal and practice objectives.

During this time we were retaining items of documentary evidence for each of the 24 indicators, e.g. extracts from the business plan and minutes of partnership meetings; sample training evaluation forms and appraisal documentation; the training policy of the practice; copies of the training plan and programme and so on.

In June 1993, seven months after making the initial commitment, we repeated the staff survey and achieved more than 80% 'yes' answers to each question. We then gathered together our documentary evidence and submitted ourselves for assessment by the TEC.

THE ASSESSMENT PROCESS

The TEC assessor initially examined the documentary evidence and then spent a day in the practice talking to partners and staff, who he selected at random. He informed us that he would be recommending us for the award. A week later, to our delight, we received confirmation that we had achieved the standard.

Case Study 40: *continued*

COSTS

The direct costs included a £500 fee for assessment. In addition, the Managing Business Change project involved a management consulting fee; £2000 of which was considered to relate directly to Investors in People and therefore met by the TEC.

The indirect costs related to the practice manager's time in putting together the documentary evidence for inspection and time invested by the whole practice at various stages on the assessment day. Time involved in actually working towards each indicator was not seen by the practice as a cost attributable to the award itself, but rather part of good management.

BENEFITS

While working towards the award we discovered previously unidentified skills throughout the practice, in particular project management skills and partners' management and organizational skills. It gave the perfect opportunity to make a thorough review of roles – partners and staff.

The role of the executive partner became more defined, together with the skills, knowledge and attributes needed to carry out the role. This gave the practice a recognized vehicle for quality improvement together with a central driving force to ensure steady progress and management change.

The practice enhanced its business plan by recognizing the training and development opportunities and implications of its objectives. By doing this we set dates and project plans. We also put ourselves in a better position to achieve those objectives by identifying skills needed and implementing training events to meet those requirements.

We developed a more open practice culture in which suggestions are welcomed and people are involved in decisions affecting their work. We reviewed, acknowledged and rewarded achievement of each group. We encouraged staff to identify new objectives to be introduced in the business plan review, thereby contributing to their ownership of the subsequent plan.

Case Study 40: *continued*

We have organized the workload more efficiently, allowing all regular practice business and meetings to take place in the normal working day.

The fear of further change has turned into a more positive attitude, whereby it is seen as an opportunity for improvement. We are able to plan effectively for changes instigated by the practice and use the skills we have learnt to ensure, wherever possible, the smooth introduction of changes imposed on the practice.

From our service standards we were readily able to produce a meaningful patient charter, the success of which has the commitment of all staff in the practice.

Possibly the most important benefit has been that, at a time of stress and demotivation generally, we have managed to lift morale and engender a sense of pride in our work, which has improved the quality of our patient care.

DIFFICULTIES

Not all staff were convinced of the benefit of training and development, but we were able to give evidence of how we were tackling this.

In a public service such as general practice it is more difficult to make a direct link to patient outcomes and quality. One example was meeting one standard in the evaluation section: 'Top management understood the broad costs and benefits of developing people'. This would be measured in a manufacturing organization as a direct link between training and improved output or quality.

We also found that monitoring service standards involved a substantial amount of measuring by audit. The time to do this was difficult to find in the early stages as there were so many standards we had not previously measured.

COMMENT

In the run-up to the assessment the whole practice, and the managers in particular, experienced a feeling of excitement and anticipation. After the euphoria of receiving the award, there was an inevitable feeling of anticlimax and to some extent a loss of direction. Motivating

Case Study 40: *continued*

ourselves to the day-to-day operation of the practice was difficult. We are allowed to retain the award for three years, after which we will be reassessed and the TEC will be looking for significant improvement.

We would probably not have considered the Investor in People award if we had not had the support of our local TEC, and the whole process would certainly have taken a lot longer had we not undertaken their 'Managing Business Change' scheme. We also received a substantial amount of support from our regional health authority. Our local FHSA was unable to support us initially but was quick to promote the practice once we had received the award.

Although there was mixed reaction from colleagues, the reaction of our patients has been extremely positive. Many of them are working towards the award in their own organizations and are aware of the standard we have reached.

One thing is certain. The practice has moved forward in terms of business planning, standard setting, implementing protocols and staff training and development. We are much more proactive, enabling us to cope better with the changes facing all of us in the NHS in the next decade.

Karen Helme, lately practice manager, Whickham Practice, Gateshead, South Tyne

CHARTERMARK

Chartermark is an award scheme for public service organizations that can demonstrate excellence in delivering of the service. The scheme was first announced in the Citizen's Charter White Paper in July 1991. Up to 100 awards can be made annually. Entrants must show the extent to which they are meeting the criteria which are set out in Box 15.1.

A helpful booklet is produced providing information about the scheme and assisting organizations prepare their applications. It is also intended to allow practices to assess the extent to which they are meeting the Chartermark criteria.

Box 15. 1   CHARTERMARK CRITERIA

1   Standards – set clear and tough performance standards and tell users about these and whether they are achieved.
2   Information and openness – tell users in a clear way about all the services available and how to access them.
3   Choice of consultation – consult users on what services they need, how they can be made better and how the practice makes use of customer ideas, where possible giving users a choice.
4   Courtesy and helpfulness – have a user friendly approach to the needs of customers.
5   Putting things right – make it easy for users to say when they are unhappy and act swiftly to put things right.
6   Value for money – budget carefully and effectively.
7   Customer satisfaction – have measures in place to identify satisfaction.
8   Measurable improvement – demonstrate improvements in service over the last two years.
9   New plan – plan to introduce one innovative improvement to service.

Applications are considered by a team of experienced Chartermark assessors, who may obtain further information from sources such as government departments. The best applications are shortlisted and visited by members of the Prime Minister's advisory panel or senior cabinet office staff, who assess what is actually taking place. All winners and shortlisted applicants receive feedback on their performance.

Case Study 41   Chartermark

BACKGROUND TO THE PRACTICE

The Ridley Medical Group is a five-partner teaching practice with approximately 13 000 patients in a relatively deprived urban area. The doctors work from a large new health centre with an attached community hospital, allowing delivery of a very comprehensive range of services.

Case Study 41: *continued*

WHY THE PRACTICE DECIDED TO APPLY FOR THE CHARTERMARK

The idea to enter the awards came from an article in *The Patient's Charter News,* circulated by the NHS Management Executive Communications Unit in January 1994. This referred to some of the aims of the Citizen's Charter to deliver what the public want – an efficient, helpful and professional service. Two of the primary health care team members separately looked at the nine criteria to see how closely the practice came to meeting them.

WHO WAS INVOLVED

Many of the members of the primary health care team had been involved in problem-solving exercises in the period before the actual application. Various quality initiatives introduced a culture of change into the practice, without which a Chartermark application would not have been successful. This was further helped by a residential team-building weekend held in October 1993 facilitated by the local FHSA.

METHOD OF WORKING

We decided to start by assessing the strengths and weaknesses of the practice, making use of SWOT analyses and staff appraisals. This allowed significant weaknesses to be identified and addressed.

Quality improvement programme

A quality improvement programme had been introduced and four members of the team were trained in problem solving by external consultants shared with the local FHSA. This group was formed into a new quality team, which developed a new telephone procedure, significantly improving service delivery and saving considerable capital expenditure by the practice.

Following the successful introduction of this procedure and in order to broaden the skills base of the practice, another new quality team was formed with two of the original team and two new members.

Repeat prescribing

The new quality team was asked by the partners to assess the problem of ordering, processing and collecting repeat prescriptions, which

Case Study 41: *continued*

was causing difficulty to staff and inconvenience to patients. This led to the introduction of a radical new repeat prescription system whereby patients phoned their request on a dedicated 'prescription hot line' and collected their medication directly from the chemist the next day.

Patient's charter

Among the agreed goals for the practice was the development of a patient's charter. Although the practice had considerable information from user surveys, it felt that more patient involvement was required. A patient participation group was formed, with doctors and reception staff nominating patients to provide a cross-section of the practice population. Six patients attended lunchtime meetings with the practice manager, two receptionists, one secretary, two nurses, one health visitor and one doctor.

This group, with help from the community health council, drafted specific standards that patients could expect as well as core standards to be monitored quarterly with the results displayed in the waiting room.

These core standards were:

- telephone answered within six rings
- routine appointments within three days
- urgent appointments on the same day
- usually no more than a 20-minute wait, or an explanation given
- repeat prescriptions ready within 24 hours on weekdays
- referral letters sent within five working days.

Complaints procedure

A multidisciplinary quality team set standards and monitored an in-house complaints procedure. A complaint was defined as 'an expression of dissatisfaction made to a staff member'.

The procedure had to be:

- accessible
- simple to operate with clear procedures and responsibilities
- speedy with time limits
- fair and confidential
- able to address all points

Case Study 41: *continued*

- able to give effective response
- audited at regular intervals to improve services.

Staff training emphasized the importance of 'getting it right' and 'putting it right' and any complaint made required that the problem be dealt with first.

All staff were trained to:

- acknowledge the complaint
- attempt to solve the problem
- if possible to give an explanation and apology before entering the practice complaints procedure.

Formal and informal procedures were drawn up with certain staff designated to deal with complaints, which were logged and used as learning experiences by everyone.

Practice leaflet

The patient group looked at the practice leaflet, as a result of which it was redesigned and rewritten to include more information on suggestions, complaints and patient charter standards.

Cellular working

Making use of SWOT analyses and staff appraisals, and after full consultation with all reception staff, a form of 'cellular working' was introduced, breaking the reception area into:

- filing
- front desk
- repeat prescriptions
- administration.

User and staff surveys have demonstrated great enthusiasm for the change to cellular working, and staff have accepted responsibility for monitoring it, meeting monthly with the practice manager to discuss problems and plan further improvements. For example, the filing team became totally responsible for all filing of notes, since which time the problem of missing notes has virtually disappeared. Front desk staff were chosen for their 'people skills', and have received further training

Case Study 41: *continued*

in communication skills and in handling aggressive patients. Staff were also designated and trained to deal with complaints.

Communications

With the introduction of the quality improvement programme a small team has been set up with one representative from each discipline; this team meets monthly to discuss its activities, and members give feedback to their own group.

Other communication tools include a quarterly newsletter copies of which are available in the waiting room, containing details of staff changes, advice about charter standards and the complaints procedure and health education features. An electronic message board, regularly updated, gives patients a wide range of advice about the services offered and how to complain. A clearly marked complaints/ suggestions box is displayed in the waiting room.

Image

Everyone was aware of the importance of promoting a good practice image. Areas targeted for staff standards included personal appearance, a suitable uniform, appropriate use of language on the telephone and face to face, smiling and eye contact, and professional behaviour. Six-monthly patient surveys, including random surveys, were carried out as required.

ASSESSMENT

The two members of the team who had separately looked at the nine criteria agreed we could demonstrate we were meeting most of these, although the value for money criterion was rather difficult to demonstrate. However, by concentrating on the effectiveness of recently introduced procedures, the introduction of skill mix, cellular working and savings made by audits, we were ultimately able to satisfy this criterion.

The application and appropriate supporting material was submitted, including specific evidence of how services were provided and what patients thought, and an assessor visited the practice. He spent about six hours looking at every aspect of our service, exploring patients' views and reviewing surveys. This assessment went forward to the judges and a few weeks later we received confirmation of the award.

Case Study 41: *continued*

COMMENT

We all know that without the selfless ·contribution of every single person any complex organization working at the sharp end of the NHS would cease to function. That contribution can be recognized in any number of ways, but all too often loyal, long-serving administrative, nursing and medical staff giving a high standard of care to a generally appreciative patient population get little more than a gift at Christmas. A commitment to introduce quality improvement can easily be given, but without a successful attitudinal and cultural change to which everyone subscribes, attempts are likely to flounder.

There is no big bang approach to Chartermark. It takes time to develop a culture of patient service and quality, with everyone committed to the common goal.

A Chartermark is awarded for three years. We found the process an excellent way of not only reviewing the quality of the service already in place, but of providing the opportunity to improve. It has helped us work with our patients, and staff to determine what is really needed.

Geoff Rawes, general practitioner, Ridley Medical Group, Blyth, Northumberland

EXTERNAL REVIEW SUMMARIZED

The six approaches to external review described here share some important characteristics. They all:

- seek to promote improvement
- use explicit standards
- seek to demonstrate compliance with these standards
- use prepared documentation as the basis of a practice survey.

There is a clear concentration on the structure and organization of a practice, and on its arrangements for patient care. Thus, for example, there is emphasis on the quality of access for patients, on the premises, the range of equipment, the presence of good systems and practice records, the ability of the practice to audit its work, and so on. These are all significant and important aspects of quality, a major step forward towards the assessment of quality as a whole.

The RCGP's Fellowship by Assessment is significantly different in that it begins with the doctor who is seeking fellowship. So, here there is also an important clinical dimension. Fellowship by Assessment tells us, for example, about a doctor's personal performance in relation to consulting, prescribing, the quality of hospital referrals, the effectiveness of clinical audit and in keeping up to date. This is a major additional benefit even though it falls short of measuring overall clinical competence.

We think that the emphasis for each approach to review places on fostering improvement is especially important, for it engenders a positive attitude to quality practice. This is revealed in practical ways. Thus, for example, trainers are offered courses and other educational activities, and have access to well-developed peer group support. Both GPQA and KOFA involve preliminary training activities and assessments as part of a developmental, formative process. And certainly some faculties of the RCGP provide active support and practical assistance for members attempting Fellowship by Assessment. Investors in People and Chartermark, being competitive awards, are in a somewhat different category, although here, too, active development is clearly encouraged. This way of combining standard setting and assessment with practical help to achievement is another important and positive dimension to quality assurance in which British general practice is showing that it can lead the way in the NHS.

It would seem that practices think that they get value for money. And regional post-graduate organizations and FHSAs and health boards feel that the investment on their part is a relatively economical way of securing practice development, quality assurance and improvement, as evidenced by the fact that the number of health authorities offering whole or part sponsorship appears to be rising steadily.

Finally, a word about the practices themselves. Practices such as we have described would appear to thrive on external review. Some, having done one kind of accreditation, are ready to move on to try another! We think the reason is that they are already confident of the quality of what they are doing, that they are already, by their own efforts, operating at a reasonably sophisticated level. External review provided the stimulus to go that extra mile, but they probably knew that they had the necessary skill, commitment and basic organization to get there. Hence their linking of external review with improving the practice.

If we are right then there is an important consequence here for the professional bodies and health commissions concerned with helping other practices to move forward. In terms of practice development, the emphasis may be most productive if focused on practices that want to succeed, but which do not yet have the basic culture and organization needed for the cycle of systematic improvement, fuelled by external review, to become self-sustaining. This must be one of the potentially most productive lines to explore for the many health commissions that are wondering how to target their efforts to give the best results. Thus, diagnostic consultancy, teambuilding support, strengthening of practice management, building up of internal clinical audit – these are the kinds of areas where health authorities can be most helpful.

So, credit should be given to the accrediting organizations and many practices that are doing this pioneering work for patients and for the professions in primary health care. And credit too, to the professional bodies, postgraduate organizations and health authorities which are underpinning and supporting these efforts, and making participation financially possible.

REFERENCES

1 Joint Committee on Postgraduate Training for General Practice (1992) *Accreditation of Regions and Schemes for Vocational Training in General Practice*. London: JCPTGP.

2 Royal College of General Practitioners (1990) *Fellowship by Assessment*. Occasional Paper 50. London: RCGP.

3 Royal College of General Practitioners (1985) What sort of doctor? Report from General Practice 23. London: RCGP.

4 King's Fund Organisational Audit (1993) *Primary Care Project*. London: King Edward VII Hospital Fund for London.

5 Medical Protection Society (1993) *General Practice Quality Assured (GPQA)*. London: MPS.

16

And in conclusion

Modern general practice is a huge subject. In this book we have had to be selective. We have been broad brush here, detailed there, and have emphasized some parts and only sketched in others.

What has become clearer than ever, especially in distilling the essence of the experiences of the many practices we have known, is the extraordinary extent to which modern practice can combine personal and community care. It is almost tailor-made for the new millennium – provided, that is, that the quality of care is right.

In closing, there are five features which for us seem to characterize the practice of quality. These are:

1   the cohesive practice. The idea that people in a complex organization can knit themselves together as a cohesive entity, and that the whole can be so much greater than the sum of the individual parts, is still very new. However, there are substantial benefits, not least in the confidence and high morale that flows from belonging to a practice which is in control of its own destiny, and knows where it is going and how to get there
2   leadership and commitment. The coherent practice must have a strong sense of commitment. Leadership will shine through in all sorts of ways. Purposeful practices are acutely aware of the world in which they have to work, and are prepared to try new ideas, or to try doing old things in new ways. The 'can do' philosophy will prevail
3   values and standards. All health professionals pride themselves on the values and standards which characterize the disciplines to which they belong. But one of the outstanding features of a practice of quality will be the way it develops its individual practice values and standards. It will bring together different disciplines and weave them into a distinctive and

increasingly explicit understanding of what 'our practice' is. These shared values and standards will provide a new and more secure foundation for learning, and for assuring competence and performance, because of the strong sense of ownership that goes with them

4   capacity to implement. Many practices have good intentions frustrated by an inability – for whatever reason – to follow through. Successful implementation is rooted in general managerial competence, which is why we have devoted so much space to this in the book. Without it, there can be no modern practice of quality

5   willingness to test against others. The practice of quality tests itself against others, to find out where it stands, whether its judgement of itself is accurate, understated or overconfident. This testing is directed at and inspired by the desire to be at the leading edge. The principle of external review is therefore an important ingredient in constantly improving quality.

In our book we have seen that many practices are already thinking and behaving along these lines. They are all leaders, all practices of quality.

No wonder we are unrepentant optimists for the future of this kind of general practice in Britain!

FURTHER READING

Berwick D M, Enthoven A, Bunker J P (1992) Quality management in the NHS: the doctor's role 1. *British Medical Journal*; **304**: 253–9.

Donabedian A (1966) Evaluating the quality of medical care. *Milbank Memorial Fund Quarterly*; **44**: 166–203.

Donaldson L (1995) Conflict, power, negotiation. *British Medical Journal*; **10**: 104–7.

Field M S, Lohr K N (1992) *Guidelines for Clinical Practice: From Development to Use*. Washington DC: National Academy Press.

Grol R, Lawrence M (1995) Quality improvement by peer review. *Oxford General Practice Series: 32*. Oxford: OUP.

Handy C (1994) *The Empty Raincoat*. London: Hutchinson.

Handy C (1989) *The Age of Unreason*. London: Business Books.

Hopkins A, Gabbey S, Neuberger J (1994) Role of users in health care in achieving a quality service. *Quality in Health Care*; **3**: 203–9.

Irvine D H (1990) *Managing for Quality in General Practice*. London: King's Fund.

Irvine D H and Irvine S (1991) *Making Sense of Audit*. Oxford: Radcliffe Medical Press.

Irvine S (1992) *Balancing Dreams and Discipline*. London: RCGP.

Maxwell R J (1992) Dimensions of quality revisited: from thought to action. *Quality in Health Care*; **1**: 171–7.

McClelland D C, Burnham D H (1976) Power is the great motivator. *Harvard Business Review*; March/April: 126–39.

Morgan G (1986) *Images of Organisation*. London: Sage.

Ovreteit J (1992) *Health Service Quality*. Oxford: Blackwell.

Pringle M, Bradly C P, Carmichael C M *et al.* (1995) Significant event auditing. A study of the feasibility and potential of case-based audits in primary medical care. *Occasional Paper 70*. London: RCGP.

Pugh D S (1990) (ed.) *Organisational Theory – selected readings*. London: Penguin Books.

Royal College of General Practitioners (1985) Quality in General Practice. *Policy Statement 2*. London: RCGP.

Royal College of General Practitioners (1995) *The development and implementation of clinical guidelines*. Report from General Practice No 26. London: RCGP.

Index